DRUGS OF CHOICE
FROM
THE MEDICAL LETTER

Published by

The Medical Letter, Inc.
1000 Main Street
New Rochelle, New York 10801-7537

800-211-2769

www.medletter.com

Copyright 2001
(ISSN 1065-6596)
The Medical Letter, Inc.
1000 Main Street
New Rochelle, New York 10801-7537

CONTENTS

EDITOR:
Mark Abramowicz, M.D.

DEPUTY EDITOR:
Gianna Zuccotti, M.D., M.P.H.

CONSULTING EDITOR:
Martin A. Rizack, M.D., Ph.D., *Rockefeller University*

ASSOCIATE EDITORS:
Donna Goodstein
Amy Faucard

CONTRIBUTING EDITORS:
Philip D. Hansten, Pharm. D., *University of Washington*
Neal H. Steigbigel, M.D., *Albert Einstein College of Medicine*

EDITORIAL ADVISORY BOARD:
William T. Beaver, M.D.,
  Georgetown University School of Medicine
Jules Hirsch, M.D.,
  Rockefeller University
James D. Kenney, M.D.,
  Yale University School of Medicine
Gerhard Levy, Pharm. D.,
  State University of NY at Buffalo, College of Pharmacy
Gerald L. Mandell, M.D.,
  University of Virginia School of Medicine
Hans Meinertz, M.D.,
  University Hospital, Copenhagen
Dan M. Roden, M.D.,
  Vanderbilt School of Medicine
F. Estelle R. Simons, M.D.,
  University of Manitoba

PUBLISHER:
Doris Peter, Ph.D.

DRUGS FOR RHEUMATOID ARTHRITIS

Many different drugs are now used to treat rheumatoid arthritis. Nonsteroidal anti-inflammatory drugs (NSAIDs), listed in the table on page 16, have analgesic and anti-inflammatory effects, but may not affect the disease process. The "disease-modifying" anti-rheumatic drugs (DMARDs) listed on page 18 have no immediate analgesic effects, but can control symptoms and may delay progression of the disease. Interactions of anti-rheumatic drugs with other drugs are listed in *The Medical Letter Handbook of Adverse Drug Interactions*, 2001.

NSAIDS — No NSAID is consistently more effective than any other, but some patients who do not respond to or tolerate one drug may respond to or tolerate another. Aspirin in high doses is as effective as any other NSAID, but may have more gastrointestinal toxicity.

Mechanism of Action — The anti-inflammatory effect of NSAIDs is due mainly to inhibition of the two isoforms of cyclooxygenase, COX-1 and COX-2. COX-1 is expressed in most tissues and is thought to protect the gastric mucosa. COX-2 is expressed in the kidney and brain and its expression can be induced in the ovary, uterus, cartilage and bone, and at sites of inflammation. Inhibition of COX-1 decreases synthesis of thromboxane in platelets and interferes with their aggregation. Inhibition of COX-2 decreases synthesis of prostacyclin in endothelium and may have a prothrombotic effect (BF McAdam et al, Proc Natl Acad Sci USA 1999; 96:272). Older NSAIDs, in varying degrees, block both COX isoforms. Celecoxib (*Celebrex* – Medical Letter 1999; 41:11) and rofecoxib (*Vioxx* – Medical Letter 1999; 41:59) in therapeutic doses selectively inhibit COX-2 but not COX-1.

Gastrointestinal Adverse Effects – All NSAIDs can cause dyspepsia and more serious gastrointestinal (GI) toxicity, including gastric and duodenal ulceration, perforation and bleeding, with or without warning symptoms in any age group, but especially among elderly patients. Meclofenamate may cause a high incidence of diarrhea. Piroxicam, which has a longer half-life, should be avoided in elderly patients. Concurrent use of misoprostol *(Cytotec)*, a prostaglandin analog, or possibly a histamine H_2-receptor antagonist such as famotidine *(Pepcid)* in high doses or a proton pump inhibitor such as omeprazole *(Prilosec)*, may decrease the incidence of GI toxicity caused by NSAIDs (P Schoenfeld et al, Aliment Pharmacol Ther 1999; 13:1273).

Celecoxib and rofecoxib have less upper GI toxicity than older, less selective NSAIDs, at least in the short term (one year or less) in patients not taking aspirin for cardiovascular prophylaxis (DR Lichtenstein and MM Wolfe, JAMA 2000; 284:1297). In a randomized, double-blind trial in almost 8000 patients with osteoarthritis or rheumatoid arthritis, celecoxib 400 mg b.i.d. (higher than recommended for any indication) was associated with fewer symptomatic ulcers or upper GI complications than ibuprofen 800 mg t.i.d. or diclofenac 75 mg b.i.d. In patients also taking aspirin, however, the incidence of GI toxicity was similar with either celecoxib or the older NSAIDs (FR Silverstein et al, JAMA 2000; 284:1247). With rofecoxib 50 mg daily, 2.1 confirmed GI events occurred per 100 patient-years, compared to 4.5 with naproxen 500 mg b.i.d. (C Bombardier et al, N Engl J Med 2000; 343:1520). Whether serious GI bleeding will occur less frequently with long-term use of celecoxib and rofecoxib than with older NSAIDs remains to be established, particularly in patients also taking cardioprotective doses of aspirin.

Effects on Bleeding and Myocardial Infarction – With the exception of nonacetylated salicylates, the selective COX-2 inhibitors and possibly meloxicam and nabumetone, all NSAIDs can interfere with platelet function and prolong bleeding time. This effect is reversible when the drug is cleared, except with aspirin. Use of selective COX-2 inhibitors, which do not interfere with platelet function and decrease the antithrombotic effect of endothelial prostacyclin, could have a prothrombotic effect leading to a higher incidence of cardiovascular events. The higher incidence of myocardial infarction in some studies of patients taking celecoxib or rofecoxib (and not taking aspirin) could also be due to the loss of a cardioprotective effect provided by a non-selective NSAID. Whether myocardial infarction will occur more frequently with long-term use of celecoxib and rofecoxib than with older NSAIDs remains to be established.

Renal Toxicity – Due to inhibition of renal prostaglandins, all NSAIDs, including selective COX-2 inhibitors, decrease renal blood flow, cause fluid retention and may cause renal failure in some patients, particularly the elderly (SK Swan et al, Ann Intern Med 2000; 113:1). Diminished renal function or decreased effective intravascular volume due to diuretic therapy, cirrhosis or congestive heart failure increases the risk of NSAID renal toxicity.

CNS Toxicity – All NSAIDs can cause central-nervous-system (CNS) effects such as dizziness, anxiety, drowsiness and confusion. Indomethacin (*Indocin*, and others) may cause more severe CNS adverse effects than other NSAIDs and should be used cautiously in the elderly; depression, disorientation and, especially, severe headache occur frequently with higher doses. Tinnitus has been associated particularly with high doses of salicylates. Aseptic meningitis has occurred rarely in patients with systemic lupus erythematosus or other connective tissue diseases taking ibuprofen, tolmetin or sulindac and has been reported with ibuprofen and naproxen in patients without any connective tissue disease.

Hepatic and Other Toxicity – NSAIDs frequently cause small increases in aminotransferase activity; serious hepatic toxicity is rare, but occurs more frequently with diclofenac. Pancreatitis also has been reported. Cholestatic hepatitis has been reported with celecoxib, which is a sulfonamide (MV Galan et al, Ann Intern Med 2001; 134:254).

NSAIDs rarely cause blood dyscrasias; aplastic anemia has been reported with ibuprofen, fenoprofen, naproxen, indomethacin, tolmetin and piroxicam. Asthmatic patients sensitive to aspirin could develop severe bronchospasm and anaphylactoid reactions with any NSAID; nonacetylated salicylates are less likely to cause reactions in these patients, and one report suggests that selective

COX-2 inhibitors may also be less likely to do so (B Dahlén et al, N Engl J Med 2001; 344:142). Various types of dermatological toxicity have been reported with NSAIDs, including photosensitivity and toxic epidermal necrolysis. Celecoxib is contraindicated in patients allergic to sulfonamides. Use of NSAIDs by pregnant women has been associated with persistent pulmonary hypertension in their offspring (MA Alano et al, Pediatrics 2001; 107:519).

Drug Interactions – NSAIDs may interact with many drugs; they may, for example, decrease the effectiveness of diuretics, beta-blockers, ACE inhibitors and some other antihypertensive drugs, and may increase the toxicity of lithium and methotrexate (*The Medical Letter Handbook of Adverse Drug Interactions*, 2001, page 371). Celecoxib and rofecoxib can increase INR and the risk of bleeding if given with warfarin (*Coumadin*, and others); the effect is unlikely to be clinically significant, but patients should be monitored for INR changes (*The Medical Letter Handbook of Adverse Drug Interactions*, 2001, page 64).

DISEASE-MODIFYING ANTI-RHEUMATIC DRUGS (DMARDs) — Most clinicians begin therapy with a DMARD—often hydroxychloroquine or sulfasalazine for mild rheumatoid arthritis or methotrexate if the disease is more severe—in addition to an NSAID at the time of diagnosis. Most DMARDs have a slow onset of action and require regular monitoring for adverse effects.

HYDROXYCHLOROQUINE (*Plaquenil*, and others) — The antimalarial hydroxychloroquine, 200 mg twice daily, is moderately effective for mild rheumatoid arthritis and is usually well tolerated (JD Jessop et al, Br J Rheumatol 1998; 37:992). The drug's effectiveness may require three to six months to become apparent. Nausea and epigastric pain can occur, but serious adverse effects are rare. Hemolysis may occur in patients with glucose-6-phosphate dehydrogenase (G6PD) deficiency. Retinal damage has been reported, but can be avoided if vision is monitored (visual fields, color vision) at six- to twelve-month intervals, dosage is kept below 6.5 mg/kg/d, and the drug is discontinued promptly when signs of retinal toxicity first appear (GD Levy et al, Arthritis Rheum 1997; 40:1482; JA Block, Lancet 1998; 351:771).

METHOTREXATE (*Rheumatrex*, and others) — Oral methotrexate in low dosage decreases symptoms, improves the long-term outcome of rheumatoid arthritis, and is often used initially. Medical Letter consultants recommend starting with 7.5 mg once a week taken as a single dose or over 24 hours, which can be increased gradually to 15 to 25 mg once a week. The anti-rheumatic effect of low-dosage once-weekly methotrexate is often apparent within four to six weeks. Intramuscular or subcutaneous methotrexate once weekly may be helpful for patients who have adverse GI effects or lose benefit over time with oral dosage. Folic acid supplements of 1 to 4 mg per day are recommended (SL Morgan et al, BioDrugs 1997; 8:164).

Adverse Effects — In low dosage, methotrexate is often well tolerated, but may cause stomatitis, anorexia, nausea, abdominal cramps and increased aminotransferase activity, and rarely bone marrow suppression, pulmonary toxicity and hepatic fibrosis. Anorexia, nausea and vomiting are less frequent with parenteral use of the drug. Hypersensitivity pneumonitis, which can be severe, occurs in 1% to 4% of rheumatoid arthritis patients taking methotrexate and may be more common in patients with antecedent lung disease. Cutaneous necrotizing vasculitis has been reported rarely (TH Simonart et al, Clin Rheumatol 1997; 16:623). The drug is immunosuppressive; infections such as herpes zoster and *Pneumocystis carinii* have been reported to be more common in patients taking methotrexate for rheumatoid arthritis. An association has been reported between methotrexate and lymphoma, but spontaneous remission has occurred in some patients with discontinuation of the drug; cause and effect remain to be established (L Georgescu and SA Paget, Drug Saf 1999; 20:475). Most clinicians would not prescribe methotrexate for patients with pre-existing liver disease or significant alcohol use. Since the drug is eliminated primarily by renal excretion, serious toxicity is more likely in patients with diminished renal function.

Methotrexate is teratogenic and should not be given to women who are or may become pregnant. It is also an abortifacient and can decrease fertility in both men and women. Men should not take the drug, if possible, for at least three months before a planned conception. Women should not take the drug for one menstrual cycle before planned conception.

In elderly patients or others with decreased renal function, concurrent use of an NSAID, which is common, increases serum concentrations and the toxicity of methotrexate (*Medical Letter Handbook of Adverse Drug Interactions*, 2001, page 339). The risk of elevated aminotransferase activity is increased in patients taking methotrexate concurrently with leflunomide; serious liver disease has been reported (ME Weinblatt et al, Arthritis Rheum 2000; 43:2609). Trimethoprim/sulfamethoxazole (*Bactrim*, and others), trimethoprim (*Proloprim*, and others) and possibly sulfasalazine may increase bone marrow suppression due to methotrexate (A Steuer and JM Gumpel, Br J Rheumatol 1998; 37:105).

SULFASALAZINE (*Azulfidine*, and others) — Sulfasalazine is also effective for treatment of rheumatoid arthritis, but has greater toxicity than hydroxychloroquine (ME Weinblatt et al, J Rheumatol 1999; 26:2123). The usual dosage of sulfasalazine is 2 g/day. Most clinicians begin with lower doses and increase gradually to minimize adverse effects. Some clinicians increase the dose to 3 grams per day if necessary.

Adverse Effects — Nausea, anorexia and rash are fairly common with sulfasalazine. Serious reactions such as hepatitis and blood dyscrasias are rare and usually occur within the first two to three months of treatment. A lupus-like syndrome has been reported. Sperm counts may decrease, but return to normal after withdrawal of the drug. Use of enteric-coated sulfasalazine (*Azulfidine En-tabs*, and others) decreases GI toxicity. Hemolysis may occur in patients with glucose-6-phosphate dehydrogenase (G6PD) deficiency.

GOLD — Gold salts have been used for many years for treatment of severe rheumatoid arthritis and sometimes can induce a complete remission. Gold sodium thiomalate (*Aurolate*) and aurothioglucose (*Solganal*) are two injectable preparations available in the USA. An oral preparation, auranofin (*Ridaura*), is also available; it is less effective than injectable gold.

Dosage – The usual dosage of injectable gold includes a test dose of 10 mg, followed one week later by 25 mg once a week for one or two weeks, and then 50 mg weekly for up to 20 weeks, or sometimes longer if improvement continues. Response usually occurs within three to six months after starting treatment. If a response occurs, treatment intervals may be increased to every two weeks, then every three weeks, and then monthly. Most patients who respond should remain on monthly therapy; some patients may require shorter intervals. Discontinuing maintenance gold therapy may result in recurrence of arthritis that may not remit when gold is re-instituted. The dosage of auranofin is 3 mg twice a day or 6 mg once daily. If the disease does not respond within three to six months, dosage may be increased to 3 mg t.i.d. if tolerated. If the response is still unsatisfactory, the drug should be discontinued.

Adverse Effects – Many patients discontinue injectable gold because of adverse effects, particularly stomatitis, rash, proteinuria and, less commonly, leukopenia and thrombocytopenia. A complete blood count and urinalysis is recommended before each dose to detect drug-related cytopenia or proteinuria. Pruritic rash and stomatitis sometimes resolve if therapy is withheld for a few weeks and then re-started cautiously at a lower dose. Enterocolitis and aplastic anemia are rare but potentially fatal adverse effects. Interstitial pneumonitis is another rare but serious adverse effect. Gold thiomalate uncommonly causes a "nitritoid" reaction, which can be severe, characterized by flushing, weakness, nausea and dizziness within 30 minutes of injection. These reactions rarely occur with aurothioglucose. Oral gold causes less mucocutaneous, bone marrow and renal toxicity than injectable gold, but more diarrhea and other GI reactions. Gold therapy is not recommended for use during pregnancy.

LEFLUNOMIDE *(Arava)* – An oral pyrimidine synthesis inhibitor (Medical Letter 1998; 40:110), leflunomide in 6- to 12-month clinical trials was as effective as methotrexate or sulfasalazine in decreasing signs and symptoms and slowing radiologic progression of rheumatoid arthritis (JS Smolen et al, Lancet 1999; 353:259; V Strand et al, Arch Intern Med 1999; 159:2542; JT Sharp et al,

Arthritis Rheum 2000; 43:495). Long-term data are not available. After a loading dose of 100 mg daily for three days, the maintenance dose is 20 mg daily; if not well tolerated, it can be reduced to 10 mg daily.

Adverse Effects – Diarrhea occurs frequently. Reversible alopecia, rash and increases in aminotransferase activity can occur, and patients should be monitored for hepatic toxicity. Anaphylaxis, Stevens-Johnson syndrome and leucocytoclastic vasculitis have been reported. Leflunomide is carcinogenic and teratogenic in animals and contraindicated during pregnancy. Women who want to become pregnant and men who want to father a child after beginning treatment with the drug should first discontinue it and take cholestyramine (*Questran*, and others) 8 grams t.i.d. for 11 days to bind and eliminate the drug; women should then verify that plasma levels of the metabolite are <0.02 mg/L. Without cholestyramine, it could take up to two years for serum concentrations of the drug to become undetectable. The active metabolite of leflunomide inhibits CYP2C9 and can lead to increases in serum concentrations of many drugs, including some NSAIDs. Combining leflunomide with methotrexate increases the risk of elevated aminotransferase activity.

AZATHIOPRINE *(Imuran,* and others) — Azathioprine, a purine analog immunosuppressive drug, given in a dosage of 1 to 2.5 mg/kg/day can also be effective for refractory rheumatoid arthritis, but some patients cannot tolerate it (CR Yates et al, Ann Intern Med 1997; 126:608; K Gaffney and DGI Scott, Br J Rheumatol 1998; 37:824).

Adverse Effects — Nausea, vomiting, abdominal pain, hepatitis and reversible bone marrow depression can occur with azathioprine. An increased risk of lymphoma has been reported. Concurrent use of allopurinol (*Zyloprim*, and others) seriously increases azathioprine toxicity and dosage adjustment is necessary (*Medical Letter Handbook of Adverse Drug Interactions*, 2001 page 25). Azathioprine is not recommended for use during pregnancy.

TUMOR NECROSIS FACTOR (TNF) INHIBITORS — Two injectable drugs that bind to and block the activity of TNF are also used to treat rheumatoid arthritis (Medical Letter 1998; 40:110; DA Fox, Arch Intern Med 2000; 160:437). TNF, a cytokine that causes inflammation, is present in the synovium and leads to recruitment of inflammatory cells, neoangiogenesis and joint destruction (EHS Choy and GS Panayi, N Engl J Med 2001; 344:907). **Etanercept** *(Enbrel)*, given subcutaneously, is a recombinant version of the soluble human TNF receptor. **Infliximab** *(Remicade)*, given intravenously, is a chimeric human/mouse anti-TNF monoclonal antibody (Medical Letter 1999; 41:19; B Jarvis and D Faulds, Drugs 1999; 57:945).

In patients who had failed to respond adequately to methotrexate alone, addition of **etanercept**, 25 mg twice a week for four months, was more effective than placebo in improving signs and symptoms of rheumatoid arthritis (ME Weinblatt et al, N Engl J Med 1999; 340:253). In patients with early rheumatoid arthritis, etanercept alone was more effective than methotrexate in decreasing symptoms and slowing joint damage (JM Bathon et al, N Engl J Med 2000; 343:1586). In patients with persistently active rheumatoid arthritis **infliximab** added to methotrexate in doses of 3 or 10 mg/kg IV at four- to eight-week intervals improved symptoms and stopped progression of joint damage (PE Lipsky et al, N Engl J Med 2000; 343:1594).

Adverse Effects – Injection-site reactions are common with **etanercept**, and auto-antibodies were detectable in some patients. Demyelinating disorders, including multiple sclerosis, myelitis and optic neuritis, have been associated with use of etanercept, but cause and effect has not been established. Fatal pancytopenia has occurred rarely. Adverse effects of **infliximab** include headache, infection and infusion reactions associated with administration of the drug (fever, urticaria, dyspnea and hypotension). Some patients developed anti-infliximab or auto-antibodies, and a few patients developed anti-nuclear antibodies and a lupus-like syndrome. Combined use with immunosuppressants may decrease development of anti-infliximab antibodies. Whether long-term use of TNF inhibitors such as etanercept or infliximab could increase the incidence of other auto-immune diseases is unknown. Serious infections, including tuberculosis and sepsis, have been reported with both etanercept and infliximab; they should not be given to patients with active localized or chronic infections. Lymphoma and other malignancies have been reported in association with both drugs, but cause and effect have not been established.

CORTICOSTEROIDS — Use of corticosteroids in rheumatoid arthritis remains controversial. Prednisone 7.5 mg daily has been reported to reduce radiographic progression of disease in early rheumatoid arthritis, but rebound deterioration can occur when the dose is lowered or the drug is stopped. Many patients who have an inadequate response or are intolerant to other DMARDs benefit from 5 to 10 mg of prednisone per day or less. Low-dose prednisone may be especially useful in pregnant and elderly patients as an alternative to other DMARDs and in younger patients to control active disease temporarily until drugs with a slower onset of action can provide sufficient control. Use of corticosteroids in higher doses may be required to control severe systemic manifestations of rheumatoid arthritis, such as pericarditis or vasculitis. Intra-articular injection of a corticosteroid such as triamcinolone hexacetonide *(Aristospan)* often can relieve an acutely inflamed rheumatoid joint without systemic consequences (JA Hunter and TH Blyth, Drug Saf 1999; 21:353).

Adverse Effects — The adverse effects of systemic corticosteroids include osteoporosis, weight gain, fluid retention, cataracts, glaucoma, acceleration of atherosclerosis, avascular necrosis, poor wound healing, gastric ulcers and GI bleeding, hyperglycemia, hypertension, adrenal suppression and increased risk of infection. Even short-term corticosteroid use in low doses can cause bone loss; calcium and vitamin D supplements should be given concurrently (Medical Letter 2000; 42:29).

OTHER DRUGS — **Cyclosporine** (*Sandimmune, Neoral*, and others) alone or with methotrexate can be useful in some patients with refractory rheumatoid arthritis, but nephrotoxicity, drug interactions and cost have limited its use (JJ Cush et al, J Rheumatol 1999; 26:1176; *Medical Letter Handbook of Adverse Drug Interactions*, 2001, page 227). The antibiotic **minocycline** (*Minocin*, and others), reported to be modestly effective and well tolerated, may be useful in early disease (JR O'Dell et al, Arthritis Rheum 1999; 42:1691). **Penicillamine** *(Depen, Cuprimine)* can be effective in patients with refractory rheumatoid arthritis and may delay progression of erosions, but its toxicity may be greater than that of methotrexate or sulfasalazine, and it is used uncommonly now. **Cyclophosphamide (***Cytoxan,* and others) may be useful for treatment of severe rheumatoid vasculitis or refractory synovitis, but long-term use increases the risk of malignancy (CD Radis et al, Arthritis Rheum 1995; 38:1120).

COMBINATION THERAPY — Combination therapy may be more effective than individual drugs (JM Kremer et al, Ann Intern Med 2001; 134:695). In treatment of early rheumatoid arthritis, combination therapy with methotrexate, sulfasalazine and hydroxychloroquine, or methotrexate, sulfasalazine and prednisone (60 mg/day tapered in six weekly steps to 7.5 mg/day), was more effective than any of the individual drugs alone (T Möttönen et al, Lancet 1999; 353:1568; M Boers et al, Lancet 1997; 350:309). Clinical trials in patients with refractory rheumatoid arthritis have found that combinations of methotrexate with sulfasalazine and hydroxychloroquine, and methotrexate plus cyclosporine, were more effective than either methotrexate or the combination of sulfasalazine and hydroxychloroquine alone (JR O'Dell et al, N Engl J Med 1996; 334:1287; CM Stein et al, Arthritis Rheum 1997; 40:1843). In one small study in patients who had failed to respond to methotrexate alone, addition of leflunomide led to a response in about half (ME Weinblatt et al, Arthritis Rheum 1999; 42:1322). Addition of etanercept or infliximab has also been effective in patients with symptoms refractory to methotrexate alone.

PLASMAPHERESIS — Limited data suggest that plasmapheresis through a protein-A-containing column (*Prosorba* – Medical Letter 1999; 41:69) that adsorbs antibodies and circulating immune complexes may decrease symptoms in 30% to 40% of patients with severe refractory rheumatoid arthritis (RM Gendreau et al, Ther Apher 2001; 5:79). The optimal number of treatments, long-term effectiveness and safety of this approach are unknown.

CONCLUSION — Most Medical Letter consultants now begin treatment of rheumatoid arthritis with both an NSAID and a disease-modifying anti-rheumatic drug (DMARD). COX-2 inhibitors have generally replaced older NSAIDs because they are less likely to cause gastrointestinal toxicity in patients not taking aspirin. Hydroxychloroquine is recommended for patients with mild arthritis and methotrexate is the DMARD of choice for moderate or severe disease. Sulfasalazine is an alternative to either drug. Combination regimens are useful in patients with symptoms refractory to initial therapy. The long-term safety and role of the new tumor-necrosis-factor inhibitors remains to be established.

COST OF SOME NONSTEROIDAL ANTI-INFLAMMATORY DRUGS

Drug	Usual dosage range for arthritis	Cost[1]
Salicylates, acetylated		
Aspirin, extended-release –	800 mg qid	
average generic price		$ 26.40
ZORprin (Knoll)		100.80
Aspirin, enteric-coated[2] –	975 mg qid	
average generic price		18.00
Ecotrin[2]		46.80
Salicylates, non-acetylated		
Choline magnesium trisalicylate –	3 grams/day in	
average generic price	1, 2 or 3 doses	52.80
Trilisate (Purdue Frederick)[3]		128.40
Sodium salicylate[2] –	3.6 to 5.4 grams/day	
average generic price	in divided doses	6.06[4]
Salicylsalicylic acid (salsalate) –	3 to 4 grams/day	
average generic price	in 2 or 3 doses	27.60
Disalcid (3M)		93.60
Mono-Gesic (Schwarz Pharma)		38.40
Celecoxib– Celebrex (Pharmacia)[3]	100 to 200 mg bid	87.60
Diclofenac – average generic price	150 to 200 mg/day	46.20
Voltaren (Novartis)	in 2 or 3 doses	96.60
Arthrotec (Pharmacia)	50 mg diclofenac + 200 µg misoprostol tid-qid	134.10
extended-release –	100 mg once/day	
average generic price		77.10
Voltaren XR		94.50
Diflunisal – average generic price	500 to 1000 mg/day in 2 doses	38.40
Dolobid (Merck)		68.40
Etodolac – average generic price	300 mg bid-tid	48.00
Lodine (Wyeth-Ayerst)		94.20
Lodine XL	400 mg once/day	45.60
Fenoprofen – average generic price	300 to 600 mg tid-qid	27.00
Nalfon (Dista)		43.20

Drug	Usual dosage range for arthritis	Cost[1]
Flurbiprofen – average generic price	200 to 300 mg/day in 2, 3 or 4 doses	$ 40.20
Ansaid (Pharmacia)		111.60
Ibuprofen[3,5] – generic price	1200 to 3200 mg/day in 3 or 4 doses	15.30
Motrin IB (McNeil)		27.00
Indomethacin[3] – average generic price	25 to 50 mg tid-qid	20.70
Indocin (Merck)		59.40
extended-release – average generic price	75 mg once/day or bid	31.20
Indocin SR (Merck)		57.30
Ketoprofen[5] – average generic price	50 mg qid or 75 mg tid	69.60
Orudis (Wyeth-Ayerst)		141.60
extended-release – average generic price	200 mg once/day	65.10
Oruvail (Wyeth-Ayerst)		89.10
Meclofenamate sodium – average generic price	200 to 400 mg/day in 3 or 4 doses	196.80
Meloxicam[6] – Mobic (Boehringer Ingelheim)	7.5 to 15 mg/day	58.80
Nabumetone – Relafen (GlaxoSmithKline)	1000 mg once/day to 2000 mg/day	76.20
Naproxen – average generic price	250 to 500 mg bid-tid	22.80
Naprosyn (Roche)[3]		60.00
enteric coated – average generic price	375 mg or 500 mg bid	49.80
EC-Naprosyn		72.00
Naproxen sodium[5] – average generic price	275 mg or 550 mg bid	25.80
Anaprox (Roche)		59.40
Oxaprozin – average generic price	600 mg once/day to 1800 mg/day	39.90
Daypro (Pharmacia)		47.70
Piroxicam – average generic price	20 mg once/day	33.30
Feldene (Pfizer)		87.60
Rofecoxib[3,6] – Vioxx (Merck)	25 to 50 mg once/day	76.20
Sulindac – average generic price	150 to 200 mg bid	29.40
Clinoril (Merck)		68.40
Tolmetin – average generic price	600 to 1800 mg/day in 3 or 4 doses	47.70
Tolectin (Ortho McNeil)		77.40[7]

1. Average cost to the patient for 30 days' treatment with the lowest recommended dosage, based on data from retail pharmacies nationwide provided by Scott-Levin's *Source[fM] Prescription Audit (SPA)*, May 2000 to April 2001.
2. Available without a prescription.
3. Also available as a liquid formulation.
4. Based on AWP price listings in *Drug Topics Red Book* 2001.
5. Also available without a prescription in a lower tablet strength.
6. Not approved for rheumatoid arthritis.
7. Based on the cost of 60 capsules of the lowest available strength.

COST OF SOME DISEASE-MODIFYING ANTI-RHEUMATIC DRUGS

Drug	Usual dosage range for arthritis	Cost[1]
Hydroxychloroquine sulfate–	200 to 400 mg/day	
average generic price		$ 25.20
Plaquenil (Sanofi Winthrop)		45.30
Methotrexate, oral –	10 to 25 mg/week	
average generic price		36.16
Rheumatrex (Lederle)		73.76
Methotrexate, injectable	10 to 25 mg/week	11.20[2]
Sulfasalazine – average generic price	2 to 3 grams/day	22.80
Azulfidine (Pharmacia & Upjohn)		37.20
enteric coated – average generic price		25.20
Azulfidine En-tabs		44.40
Gold Salts		
Gold sodium thiomalate –	50 mg/week	
Aurolate (Taylor)		45.48
Aurothioglucose – *Solganal*	50 mg/week	61.72
(Schering)		
Auranofin – *Ridaura* (Connetics)	3 mg bid or 6 mg once	136.80
Leflunomide – *Arava* (Aventis)	20 mg/day	242.10[3]
Azathioprine – average generic price	2.5 mg/kg/day	128.40
Imuran (Faro)		181.20[4]
Etanercept – *Enbrel* (Immunex)	25 mg, 2 times/week	1,062.80
Infliximab – *Remicade* (Centocor)	3 mg/kg at 0, 2 and	1,282.56[5]
	6 wks, then every 8 weeks	
Cyclosporine, oral	2.5 to 4 mg/kg/day	
average generic price[6]		270.30
Sandimmune (Novartis)		341.70[6]
microemulsion – average generic price[6]		276.90
Neoral (Novartis)		303.30[6]
Minocycline – average generic price	50 to 200 mg/day	24.60
Minocin (Lederle)		63.60
Penicillamine – *Cuprimine* (Merck)	500 to 750 mg/day	63.60
Depen (Wallace)		138.60

1. Average cost to the patient for 30 days' or 4 weeks' treatment with the lowest recommended dosage, based on data from retail pharmacies nationwide provided by Scott-Levin's *Source*™ *Prescription Audit (SPA)*, May 2000 to April 2001.
2. Average cost of one 25-mg vial per week.
3. Cost based on 30 days at 20 mg/day. The manufacturer recommends a loading dose of 100 mg/day for the first three days.
4. Cost based on purchase of 120 50-mg tablets.
5. Cost of two 100-mg vials, one dose for a 65-kg patient.
6. Cost for a 70-kg patient.

DRUGS FOR ASTHMA

Asthma is a chronic inflammatory disorder of the airways; inflammation caused by allergens, viral respiratory infections or other stimuli leads to bronchial hyperresponsiveness and obstruction of airflow (WW Busse and RF Lemanske Jr, N Engl J Med 2001; 344:350). Anti-inflammatory drugs, particularly inhaled corticosteroids, are central to its management. Treatment of asthma in the hospital or emergency department is not addressed here.

INHALATION DELIVERY DEVICES — Delivery devices, drug formulation and patient technique determine the doses of inhaled drugs that reach the lung (HW Kelly, Respir Care Clin N Am 1999; 5:537; AM Wilson et al, Lancet 1999; 353:2128). Inhaled drugs for asthma have been available in the USA mainly in pressurized metered-dose inhalers, which require a propellant. The chlorofluorocarbon (CFC) propellants in these formulations are being changed for environmental reasons, usually to hydrofluoroalkanes (HFA) (JG Goldin et al, J Allergy Clin Immunol 1999; 104:S258). Dry-powder inhalers, which are activated by inspiration, do not require a propellant, and patients who have difficulty with hand-breath coordination find them easier to use. Some young children and elderly patients may be unable to activate a dry-powder inhaler and may need to use a metered-dose inhaler with a spacer device or a nebulizer.

BETA$_2$ AGONISTS — Inhaled short-acting beta$_2$-adrenergic agonists are the most effective drugs available for treatment of acute bronchospasm and for prevention of exercise-induced asthma. Regular use of short-acting beta$_2$ agonists offers no advantage over PRN use. Levalbuterol, the R-isomer of racemic albuterol, offers no clinically significant advantage over racemic albuterol (Medical Letter 1999; 41:51; MJ Asmus and L Hendeles, Pharmacotherapy 2000; 20:123).

Long-acting beta$_2$ agonists have a prolonged effect that may last 12 hours. Salmeterol *(Serevent)* has a slower onset of action (10 to 12 minutes) compared to one to three minutes with formoterol *(Foradil* – Medical Letter 2001; 43:39). Patients taking either one of them regularly should use a short-acting beta$_2$ agonist PRN to control acute symptoms. Twice-daily inhalation of a long-acting beta$_2$ agonist in combination with an inhaled corticosteroid has been effective for maintenance treatment and may be especially useful in patients with nocturnal symptoms. In moderate asthma, addition of a long-acting beta$_2$ agonist to an inhaled corticosteroid may be more effective than raising the dose of the corticosteroid (JJ Condemi et al, Ann Allergy Asthma Immunol 1999; 82:383; RA Pauwels et al, N Engl J Med 1997; 337:1045; JA van Noord et al, Thorax 1999; 54:207). A product that combines both salmeterol and the corticosteroid fluticasone in a dry powder formulation *(Advair Diskus)* is now available (Medical Letter 2001; 43:31).

Regular use of either salmeterol or formoterol may result in tolerance to the bronchoprotective effect and mask signs of increasing inflammation (DH Yates et al, Am J Respir Crit Care Med 1995; 152:7170; RA McIvor et al, Am J Respir Crit Care Med 1998; 158:924). Long-acting beta$_2$ agonists should not be used as monotherapy; they should always be taken concurrently with an inhaled corticosteroid (SC Lazarus et al, JAMA 2001; 285:2583; RF Lemanske, Jr et al, JAMA 2001; 285:2594).

Oral beta$_2$ agonists have a slower onset of action and greater risk of adverse effects than the same drugs given by inhalation. Extended-release products given q12h may be beneficial in adults unable to use a metered-dose inhaler correctly and for nocturnal asthma. Oral syrup formulations may be useful for some young children and elderly patients with infrequent mild symptoms who cannot use an inhaler and spacer device.

Adverse Effects – Albuterol, bitolterol, pirbuterol, terbutaline, salmeterol and formoterol are relatively beta$_2$-selective in their action and produce more bronchodilation with fewer cardiovascular effects than older adrenergic drugs such as epinephrine, isoproterenol or metaproterenol. Nevertheless, tachycardia, palpitations, tremor and paradoxical bronchospasm can occur, and high doses can cause hypokalemia. Overuse of inhaled beta$_2$ agonists has been associated with an increase in mortality, probably due to failure to treat the underlying inflammation with corticosteroids. Beta-adrenergic blockers such as propranolol (*Inderal*, and others) taken concurrently decrease the bronchodilating effect of beta-adrenergic agonists.

COST OF SOME DRUGS FOR ASTHMA

Drug	Formulation	Adult Dosage	Pediatric Dosage[1]	Cost[2]
Inhaled beta$_2$-adrenergic agonists, short-acting				
Albuterol[3] –	metered-dose in-	2 puffs q4-6h	2 puffs q4-6h	
generic price (HCFA)	haler (90 µg/puff)	PRN	PRN	$ 5.93
Proventil (Schering)				33.48
Proventil HFA (non-CFC propellant)				32.57
Ventolin (GlaxoSmithKline)				32.77
Ventolin Rotacaps	dry-powder in-haler (200 µg/ inhalation)	1-2 capsules q4-6h PRN	1-2 capsules q4-6h PRN	37.92
Albuterol sulfate[3]	nebulized	2.5 mg q4-6h	0.1-0.15mg/kg	
generic price (HCFA)	(5 mg/ml)	PRN	q4-6h PRN	
single-dose vials				60.00
multi-dose vials				16.65
Proventil (Schering)				
single-dose vials				195.28
multi-dose vials				53.53
Ventolin (GlaxoSmithKline)				
multi-dose vials				51.80
		(continued)		

1. Less than 40 kg.
2. Cost of short-acting beta-adrenergic drugs is based on the cost of 100 doses. Cost of other drugs is based on 30 days' treatment with the lowest recommended adult dosage, according to AWP or HCFA listings in *Drug Topics Red Book* 2001 and June *Update* and *First DataBank PriceAlert*, June 15, 2001.

Drug	Formulation	Adult Dosage	Pediatric Dosage[1]	Cost[2]
Inhaled beta$_2$-adrenergic agonists, short-acting *(continued)*				
Levalbuterol – *Xopenex* (Sepracor)	nebulized (0.63 or 1.25 mg/3ml)	0.63 mg q6-8h PRN	Not approved	$208.00
Bitolterol mesylate[3] – *Tornalate* (Dura)	nebulized (2 mg/ml)	1.5-3.5 mg bid-qid PRN	1.5 mg bid-qid PRN	39.18
Pirbuterol – *Maxair* (3M)	metered-dose inhaler (200 µg/puff)	2 puffs q4-6h PRN	2 puffs q4-6h PRN	31.20
Maxair Autohaler	breath-actuated metered-dose inhaler (200µg/puff)	2 puffs q4-6h PRN	2 puffs q4-6h PRN	30.14
Inhaled beta$_2$-adrenergic agonist, long-acting				
Formoterol – *Foradil* (Novartis)	dry-powder inhaler (12 µg/inhalation)	1 inhalation q12h	1 inhalation q12h	70.08
Salmeterol – *Serevent* (GlaxoSmithKline)	metered-dose inhaler (21 µg/puff)	2 puffs q12h	1-2 puffs q12h	73.00
Serevent Diskus	dry-powder inhaler (50 µg/inhalation)	1 inhalation q12h	1 inhalation q12h	76.20
Salmeterol/fluticasone *Advair Diskus* (GlaxoSmithKline)	dry-powder inhaler (50 µg/100, 250 or 500 µg per inhalation	1 inhalation q12h		103.94
Oral beta$_2$-adrenergic agonists, extended release				
Albuterol sulfate – *Proventil Repetabs* (Schering)	extended-release tablets (4-mg or 8-mg tablets)	4-8 mg q12h	4 mg q12h	50.14
Volmax (Muro)				52.34

3. Nebulized solutions may be more convenient for very young, very old and other patients unable to use pressurized aerosols, and higher drug doses can be used. More time is required to administer the drug, however, and the device is usually not portable.

Drug	Formulation	Adult Dosage	Pediatric Dosage[1]	Cost[2]
Inhaled Corticosteroids				
Beclomethasone dipropionate –	metered-dose inhaler			
Vanceril (Schering)	(42 µg/puff)	4-8 puffs bid	2-4 puffs bid	$52.63
Vanceril Double-Strength (Schering)	(84 µg/puff)	2-4 puffs bid	1-2 puffs bid	53.33
QVAR (3M)	(40 µg/puff)	2-4 puffs bid	1-2 puffs bid	49.58
	(80 µg/puff)	1-2 puffs bid	1 puff bid	31.22
Budesonide –				
Pulmicort Turbuhaler (AstraZeneca)	dry-powder inhaler (200 µg/inhalation)	1-2 inhalations bid	1-2 inhalations bid	37.16
Pulmicort Respules	nebulized (0.25 or 0.5 mg/2 ml)		0.25-0.5 mg bid or 0.5 mg-1 mg once	126.00
Flunisolide – Aerobid (Forest)	metered-dose inhaler (250 µg/puff)	2-4 puffs bid or 4-8 puffs once/day	2 puffs bid	80.41
Fluticasone propionate – Flovent (GlaxoSmithKline)	metered-dose inhaler (44, 110 or 220 µg/puff)	2-4 puffs bid (44 µg/puff)	1-2 puffs bid (44 µg/puff)	49.30[4]
Flovent Rotadisk	dry-powder inhaler (50, 100 or 250 µg/inhalation)	1 inhalation bid (100 µg/inhalation)	1 inhalation bid (50 µg/inhalation)	51.76[4]
Triamcinolone acetonide – Azmacort (Aventis)	metered-dose inhaler (100 µg/puff)	2 puffs tid-qid or 4 puffs bid	1-2 puffs tid-qid or 2-4 puffs bid	46.65
Leukotriene Modifiers				
Montelukast[5] – Singulair (Merck)	tablets	10 mg once per day	5 mg once per day[6]	79.26
Zafirlukast[5] – Accolate (AstraZeneca)	tablets	20 mg bid	10 mg bid	64.64
Zileuton – Zyflo (Abbott)	tablets	600 mg qid	Not approved	100.48

4. For the metered-dose inhaler, cost is based on the 44 µg/puff dose. For the dry-powder inhaler, cost is based on the 100 µg/inhalation preparation.
5. Montelukast is taken once daily in the evening, with or without food. Zafirlukast is taken one hour before or two hours after a meal.
6. A 4-mg formulation is available for children 2 to 5 years old.

Drug	Formulation	Adult Dosage	Pediatric Dosage[1]	Cost[2]
Cromolyn sodium				
Intal (Aventis)	metered-dose inhaler (800 µg/puff)	2-4 puffs tid-qid	2-4 puffs tid-qid	$73.67
Nedocromil sodium				
Tilade (Aventis)	metered-dose inhaler (1.75 mg/puff)	2-4 puffs bid-qid	2-4 puffs bid or 2 puffs qid	49.29
Theophylline –				
average generic price	extended-release capsules or tablets[7]	300-600 mg/day	10 mg/kg/day[8]	4.32
Slo-Bid Gyrocaps (Aventis)				17.48
Theo-Dur (Key)				13.00
Unidur (Key)		400-600 mg/day		24.26

7. Extended-release formulations may not be interchangeable.
8. Starting dose. Usual maximum is 16 mg/kg/day in children more than 1 year old and in infants 5 mg/kg/day + 0.2 (age in weeks).

INHALED CORTICOSTEROIDS — Regular use of an inhaled corticosteroid can suppress inflammation and decrease bronchial hyperresponsiveness, symptoms and the risk of death in patients with persistent asthma (S Suissa et al, N Engl J Med 2000; 343:332). Inhaled corticosteroids are recommended for treatment of patients with mild or moderate persistent asthma as well as those with severe disease. The optimum dosage of inhaled corticosteroids, the lowest one that controls symptoms, may increase or decrease over time.

Adverse Effects – Recommended doses of inhaled corticosteroids have generally been free of serious toxicity. Dose-dependent slowing of linear growth may occur within six to 12 weeks in some children and adolescents; the effect, if any, on final adult height is uncertain (M Purucker and S Malozowski; and others, N Engl J Med 2001; 344:607). Suppression of the hypothalamic-pituitary-adrenal axis and dermal thinning can occur with high doses. Decreased bone density, glaucoma and posterior subcapsular cataract formation have been reported (CA Wong et al, Lancet 2000; 355:1399; RG Cumming and P Mitchell, Drug Saf 1999; 20:77; P Mitchell et al, Ophthalmology 1999; 106:2301). The risk of cataracts is greatest in adults more than 40 years old (SS Jick et al, Epidemiology 2001: 12:229). Cataracts were not reported in a five-year prospective study of budesonide 400 µg daily in 311 children (The Childhood Asthma Management Program Research Group, N Engl J Med 2000; 343:1054). Churg-Strauss vasculitis has been reported rarely in association with a reduction in the dosage of inhaled and oral corticosteroids.

Dysphonia and oral candidiasis can occur due to local deposition of the drug. Invasive pulmonary aspergillosis has been reported in a patient with asthma treated with high doses of inhaled fluticasone (BA Leav et al, N Engl J Med 2000; 343:586). Using a spacer device and rinsing the mouth after inhalation decrease the incidence of candidiasis.

LEUKOTRIENE MODIFIERS — Cysteinyl leukotrienes are products of arachidonic acid metabolism that promote chemotaxis of inflammatory cells (especially eosinophils), production of mucus and edema of the airway wall, and cause bronchoconstriction. Montelukast and zafirlukast are leukotriene receptor antagonists. Zileuton inhibits synthesis of leukotrienes.

Montelukast *(Singulair)* – In placebo-controlled clinical trials, montelukast has been modestly effective for maintenance treatment of adults and children with intermittent or persistent asthma (Medical Letter 1998; 40:71; B Jarvis and A Markham, Drugs 2000; 59:891). It is taken once daily in the evening, with or without food. As monotherapy it is less effective than inhaled corticosteroids, but addition of montelukast may improve asthma control and permit a reduction in corticosteroid dosage (FER Simons et al, J Pediatr 2001; 138:694; K Malmstrom et al, Ann Intern Med 1999; 130:487; C-G Löfdahl et al, BMJ 1999; 319:87). Montelukast is only partially effective in inhibiting aspirin response in patients with aspirin-intolerant asthma (DD Stevenson et al, Ann Allergy Asthma Immunol 2000; 85:477). Churg-Strauss vasculitis has been reported with use of montelukast, but in most cases could have been a consequence of corticosteroid withdrawal rather than an effect of the leukotriene modifier (ME Wechsler et al, Drug Saf 1999; 21:241; JM Tuggey and HSR Hosker, Thorax 2000; 55:805). Montelukast has fewer drug interactions than zafirlukast or zileuton.

Zafirlukast (Accolate) – Zafirlukast has been modestly effective as monotherapy for maintenance treatment of patients with mild to moderate asthma; it may be less effective in older patients (Medical Letter 1996; 38:111; CJ Dunn and KL Goa, Drugs 2001; 61:285). It is less effective than inhaled corticosteroids (ER Bleecker et al, J Allergy Clin Immunol 2000; 105:1123). Taking zafirlukast with food decreases its bioavailability; the manufacturer recommends taking it twice daily one hour before or two hours after a meal.

Severe hepatitis has been reported; one patient developed liver failure that required a transplant (JF Reinus et al, Ann Intern Med 2000; 133:964). Hepatic toxicity appears to be more common in females. Arthralgia and myalgia have occurred. Drug-induced lupus has been reported in one patient (TH Finkel et al, J Allergy Clin Immunol 1999; 103:533). Churg-Strauss vasculitis has also been reported with use of zafirlukast, but cause and effect have not been established (RL Green and AG Vayonis, Lancet 1999; 353:725; M Wechsler and JM Drazen, Lancet 1999; 353:1970).

Zafirlukast is metabolized by CYP2C9 and may interact with other drugs. In a single case report, concurrent use of zafirlukast was associated with toxic serum concentrations of theophylline (RK Katial et al, Arch Intern Med 1998; 158:1713). Theophylline given concurrently can also decrease the effect of zafirlukast. Zafirlukast increases serum concentrations of oral anticoagulants and may cause bleeding (*The Medical Letter Handbook of Adverse Drug Interactions*, 2001, page 442).

Zileuton (Zyflo) – Zileuton has been effective for maintenance treatment of asthma, but it is taken four times a day and patients must be monitored for hepatic toxicity (Medical Letter 1997; 39:18). One direct comparison with theophylline suggested that zileuton is equally effective in treating persistent asthma, but with a slower onset of action (HJ Schwartz et al, Arch Intern Med 1998; 158:141). Controlled comparisons with inhaled corticosteroids are not available. Zileuton, when added to a regimen of medium to high doses of inhaled or oral corticosteroids, led to greater control of asthma and nasal symptoms in patients with aspirin-induced asthma (B Dahlén et al, Am J Respir Crit Care Med 1998; 157:1187).

Zileuton is metabolized by the CYP1A2, 2C9 and 3A4. Given concurrently, it can decrease clearance and markedly increase serum concentrations of theophylline, and can also cause clinically significant increases in serum concentrations of warfarin (*Coumadin*, and others) and propranolol (*Inderal*, and others) (*The Medical Letter Handbook of Adverse Drug Interactions*, 2001, page 443).

CROMOLYN SODIUM *(Intal)* AND NEDOCROMIL SODIUM *(Tilade)* — Cromolyn sodium, an inhibitor of mast cell degranulation, can decrease airway hyperresponsiveness in some patients with asthma. The drug has no bronchodilating activity and is useful only for prophylaxis. A four-week trial may be necessary to determine whether it is effective. In one study, cromolyn was not significantly better than a placebo in preventing asthma symptoms and improving pulmonary function (MJA Tasche et al, Lancet 1997; 350:1060). Cromolyn has virtually no systemic toxicity. Nedocromil is a chemically unrelated drug with similar effects (Medical Letter 1993; 35:62). Some patients have complained about its taste. Both cromolyn and nedocromil are much less effective than inhaled corticosteroids (The Childhood Asthma Management Program Research Group, N Engl J Med 2000; 343:1054).

THEOPHYLLINE — Oral theophylline has a slower onset of action than inhaled beta$_2$ agonists and has limited usefulness for treatment of acute asthma symptoms. It can, however, reduce the frequency and severity of symptoms, especially in nocturnal asthma, and can decrease inhaled corticosteroid requirements (DJ Evans et al, N Engl J Med 1997; 337:1412). Since theophylline absorption and clearance vary, and the drug has a narrow therapeutic index, measurements of serum concentrations are needed to determine optimal dosage.

Adverse Effects – When theophylline is used alone, serum concentrations between 5 and 15 µg/ml are most likely to produce therapeutic results with minimal adverse effects. At higher serum concentrations of the drug, nausea, nervousness, headache and insomnia may occur. Vomiting, hypokalemia, hyperglycemia, tachycardia, cardiac arrhythmias, tremor, neuromuscular irritability and seizures can also occur. Many other drugs used concomitantly can cause either an increase or decrease in serum theophylline concentrations (*The Medical Letter Handbook of Adverse Drug Interactions*, 2001, page 428).

IPRATROPIUM — Ipratropium bromide, an inhaled anticholinergic agent available both alone *(Atrovent)* and in combination with albuterol *(Combivent)*, acts as a bronchodilator and is used to relieve bronchospasm in chronic bronchitis and chronic obstructive pulmonary disease (COPD). It is not FDA-approved for use in asthma. Ipratropium has a slower onset of action than short-acting $beta_2$ agonists, but can be used in patients unable to tolerate $beta_2$-agonists and in those who have both asthma and COPD. Dry mouth, pharyngeal irritation, urinary retention and increases in intraocular pressure may occur; the drug should be used with caution in patients with glaucoma and in those with prostatic hypertrophy or bladder neck obstruction.

ORAL CORTICOSTEROIDS — Oral corticosteroids are the most effective drugs available for acute exacerbations of asthma unresponsive to bronchodilators (S Schuh et al, N Engl J Med 2000; 343:689). Even when an acute exacerbation responds to bronchodilators, many clinicians treat recovering patients for up to 10 days with oral corticosteroids, which decrease symptoms and may prevent an early relapse (K Chapman et al, N Engl J Med 1991; 324:788). Chronic daily use of oral corticosteroids can cause glucose intolerance, weight gain, increased blood pressure, bone demineralization leading to osteoporosis, cataracts, immunosuppression and decreased linear growth in children. Alternate-day use of corticosteroids can decrease the incidence of adverse effects, but not of osteoporosis, the most common major complication of long-term use.

EXERCISE-INDUCED BRONCHOSPASM — Most patients with exercise-induced bronchospasm inhale a short-acting $beta_2$ agonist before exercise. Long-acting $beta_2$ agonists may offer protection for prolonged physical activity, but regular long-term use may decrease the duration of the bronchoprotective effect (FER Simons, Pediatrics 1997; 99:655; JA Nelson et al, N Engl J Med 1997; 339:141). In some patients, cromolyn or nedocromil taken before exercise can be effective against exercise-induced bronchospasm. Leukotriene modifiers taken regularly may decrease exercise-induced bronchospasm, but many patients show little or no response to these drugs (JP Kemp et al, J Pediatr 1998; 133:424). The US Olympic Committee allows athletes to use cromolyn, nedocromil, ipratropium, theophylline and all the leukotriene modifiers without prior approval; the inhaled beta$_2$ agonists (albuterol, terbutaline, salmeterol and formoterol) and most inhaled corticosteroids require prior approval. The National Collegiate Athletic Association (NCAA) permits most asthma medications except for oral beta$_2$ agonists.

ASTHMA DURING PREGNANCY AND LACTATION – Clinical experience suggests that many of the drugs used to treat asthma can be used safely during pregnancy and lactation (KS Tan and NC Thomson, Am J Med 2000; 109:727; Joint Committee, Ann Allergy Asthma Immunol 2000; 84:475). Among the inhaled corticosteroids, the longest experience has been with beclomethasone, but budesonide also appears to be safe (B Källen et al, Obstet Gynecol 1999; 93:392). Metaproterenol, terbutaline, albuterol, salmeterol, theophylline, cromolyn, nedocromil and ipratropium are all considered safe for use during pregnancy. Based on animal studies, montelukast and zafirlukast may be safe to use, but zileuton should be avoided. Taking theophylline during lactation may produce irritability in the newborn. Oral corticosteroids may decrease birth weight and increase the risk of pre-eclampsia, and possibly increase the risk of oral cleft defects (E Rodriguez-Pinilla and ML Martinez-Frias, Teratology 1998; 58:8); in severe asthma, however, their benefits outweigh the risks.

CHOICE OF DRUGS — Both children and adults with infrequent mild symptoms of asthma may require only intermittent use, as needed, of a short-acting inhaled beta$_2$-adrenergic agonist. Patients with exercise-induced asthma can use a beta$_2$ agonist before exercise. Overuse of inhaled short-acting beta$_2$ agonists (daily use according to some clinicians, or more than twice a week according to National Institutes of Health guidelines) indicates that an inhaled corticosteroid should be added to the treatment regimen or, if one is already being used, that the dosage should be increased. The role of leukotriene modifiers as possible alternatives to inhaled corticosteroids in mild asthma remains to be established.

Maintenance treatment with a long-acting inhaled $beta_2$ agonist such as salmeterol or formoterol in addition to an inhaled corticosteroid can control symptoms in patients with moderate or persistent asthma. Oral theophylline can also suppress the symptoms of asthma, particularly nocturnal symptoms, but requires careful titration of dosage and monitoring of serum concentrations. A five- to ten-day course of oral corticosteroids can control severe acute asthma symptoms unresponsive to other drugs.

DRUGS OF CHOICE FOR CANCER CHEMOTHERAPY

The tables that follow list drugs used for treatment of cancer in the USA and Canada and their major adverse effects. The choice of drugs in Table I is based on the opinions of Medical Letter consultants. Some drugs are listed for indications for which they have not been approved by the US Food and Drug Administration. For many of the cancers listed, surgery and/or radiation therapy are also part of the management of the disease. Anticancer drugs and their adverse effects are listed in Table II on page 41. A partial list of brand names appears on page 54.

TABLE I – DRUGS OF CHOICE

Cancer	Drugs of choice	Some alternative or additional drugs
Adrenocortical	Mitotane; Cisplatin ± etoposide	Doxorubicin Drugs for palliation of hormone hypersecretion: ketoconazole, aminoglutethimide, metyrapone
Anal	Fluorouracil + mitomycin	Cisplatin
Biliary tract	Fluorouracil ± leucovorin	Fluorouracil + doxorubicin + mitomycin (FAM); cisplatin; gemcitabine
Bladder	*Superficial:* Instillation of BCG	*Superficial:* Instillation of mitomycin, doxorubicin, thiotepa or valrubicin[1]
	Systemic: Methotrexate + vinblastine + doxorubicin + cisplatin (MVAC)	*Systemic:* Cisplatin + methotrexate + vinblastine (CMV)[2]; paclitaxel + carboplatin; gemcitabine + cisplatin; ifosfamide with mesna; gallium nitrate

1. Medical Letter 1999; 41:32
2. For patients who cannot tolerate doxorubicin.

Cancer	Drugs of choice	Some alternative or additional drugs
Brain		
anaplastic astro-cytoma/glio-blastoma	Procarbazine + lomustine + vincristine; Carmustine-containing polymer wafer	Temozolomide[3]; carmus-tine; cisplatin or carbopla-tin
anaplastic oligo-dendroglioma	Procarbazine + lomustine + vincristine	Carmustine; cisplatin
medulloblast-oma/embryonal tumors	Lomustine + cisplatin + vincristine; Vincristine + cisplatin + cyclophospha-mide + etoposide	Lomustine + vincristine + prednisone
germ cell tumors	Cisplatin or carboplatin + etoposide	Vinblastine, bleomycin, cy-clophosphamide
primary central-nervous-system lymphoma	Intravenous high-dose methotrexate ± intrathecal methotrexate; high dose intravenous cytarabine	Blood-brain-barrier disrup-tion with intravenous cy-clophosphamide, intra-arterial methotrexate + leucovorin, and oral pro-carbazine and dexametha-sone
Breast	*Risk reduction:* Tamoxifen[4] *Adjuvant*[5]: Doxorubicin + cyclophosphamide ± fluo-rouracil (AC or CAF) fol-lowed by paclitaxel; Cyclo-phosphamide + methotrex-ate + fluorouracil (CMF); Tamoxifen for receptor-positive and hormone-responsive	Cyclophosphamide + epirubicin[6] + fluorouracil (CEF)
	Metastatic: Doxorubicin + cyclophosphamide ± flu-orouracil (AC or CAF); Cy-clophosphamide + metho-trexate + fluorouracil (CMF); For receptor-positive and/or hormone-responsive: tamoxifen, toremifene, letrozole[7] or anastrazole[8]	Paclitaxel; docetaxel; capecitabine; vinorelbine; mitoxantrone; epirubicin; fluorouracil by continuous infusion For receptor-positive and/or hormone-respon-sive: exemestane[9]; meges-trol acetate; fluoxy-mesterone

---

3. Medical Letter 1999; 41:123
4. Medical Letter 1999; 41:1
5. Adjuvant treatment with chemotherapy and/or tamoxifen is generally recommend-ed for all node-positive patients, and for node-negative patients with tumors > 1 cm in size or other unfavorable prognostic features. Use of tamoxifen is limited to pa-tients with tumors that are hormone-receptor-positive or unknown. An anthracy-cline-containing regimen is preferred in patients with node-positive disease, or in patients with tumors that overexpress HER-2/Neu.

Cancer	Drugs of choice	Some alternative or additional drugs
Breast *(continued)*	For tumors overexpressing HER2 protein: Doxorubicin + cyclophosphamide + trastuzumab[10]; paclitaxel + trastuzumab	Trastuzumab
Carcinoid	Fluorouracil + streptozocin; Doxorubicin	Dacarbazine; interferon alfa For symptoms of carcinoid syndrome: octreotide
Cervix	*Locally advanced:* Cisplatin ± fluorouracil *Metastatic:* Cisplatin; Ifosfamide with mesna; Bleomycin + ifosfamide with mesna + cisplatin (BIP)	Carboplatin; fluorouracil; epirubicin; paclitaxel; doxorubicin; vinblastine; methotrexate; mitomycin; irinotecan
Choriocarcinoma	Methotrexate ± leucovorin; Dactinomycin	Etoposide + methotrexate + dactinomycin + cyclophosphamide + vincristine (EMA-CO); methotrexate + dactinomycin + cyclophosphamide (MAC); cisplatin ± etoposide
Colorectal	*Adjuvant:* Fluorouracil + leucovorin *Metastatic:* Fluorouracil + leucovorin + irinotecan[11]	Capecitabine; oxaliplatin[†]; tegafur/uracil[†] + leucovorin[12] For hepatic metastases: hepatic intra-arterial (HIA) floxuridine

† Available in the USA for investigational use only.

6. Medical Letter 2000; 42:12
7. H Mouridsen et al, J Clin Oncol 2001; 19:2596
8. J Bonneterre et al, J Clin Oncol 2000; 18:3748; JM Nabholtz et al, J Clin Oncol 2000; 18:3758
9. Medical Letter 2000; 42:35
10. DJ Slamon et al, N Engl J Med 2001; 344:783
11. Fluorouracil, leucovorin and irinotecan are generally considered the drugs of choice for treatment of metastatic colorectal cancer because improved survival has been documented with this combination, but the optimal dosage regimen is unclear (L Saltz et al, N Engl J Med 2000; 343:905; JY Douillard et al, Lancet 2000; 355:1041, 1372). A higher-than-expected mortality rate in the first 60 days of treatment has been reported in some patients treated with these drugs (DJ Sargent et al, N Engl J Med 2001; 345:144).
12. R Pazdur et al, Proc Am Soc Clin Oncol 1999; 18:263a, abstract 1009.

Cancer	Drugs of choice	Some alternative or additional drugs
Endometrial	Doxorubicin + cisplatin ± cyclophosphamide; Megestrol or another progestin	Epirubicin; tamoxifen; carboplatin; paclitaxel
Esophageal	Cisplatin + fluorouracil	Paclitaxel; doxorubicin; methotrexate; vinorelbine; bleomycin; irinotecan
Ewing's sarcoma (Also Primitive neuroectodermal tumor)	Vincristine + doxorubicin + cyclophosphamide alternating with ifosfamide with mesna + etoposide	Dactinomycin
Gastric	Fluorouracil ± leucovorin	Fluorouracil + doxorubicin + methotrexate (FAMTX) or mitomycin (FAM); infusional fluorouracil + cisplatin; etoposide; paclitaxel; docetaxel; irinotecan + cisplatin
Head and neck[13]	Cisplatin + fluorouracil or paclitaxel	Docetaxel; methotrexate; bleomycin; carboplatin; ifosfamide
Hepatoblastoma	Vincristine + cisplatin + fluorouracil; Cisplatin + doxorubicin	Etoposide; carboplatin; ifosfamide with mesna
Islet cell	Streptozocin + doxorubicin	Streptozocin + fluorouracil; chlorozotocin[†]; dacarbazine; interferon alfa For symptomatic relief: octreotide
Kaposi's sarcoma	Liposomal doxorubicin or daunorubicin; Doxorubicin + bleomycin + vincristine (ABV)	Vinblastine; etoposide; interferon alfa; paclitaxel; vinorelbine; alitretinoin gel
Leukemia		
Acute lymphocytic leukemia (ALL)	*Induction:* Vincristine + prednisone + asparaginase + daunorubicin or doxorubicin ± cyclophosphamide *CNS prophylaxis:* Intrathecal methotrexate (± intrathecal cytarabine ± intrathecal hydrocortisone) ± systemic high-dose methotrexate with leucovorin	*Induction:* Same ± high-dose methotrexate ± cytarabine; pegaspargase substitution for asparaginase; teniposide or etoposide; high-dose cytarabine + mitoxantrone; ifosfamide with mesna

Cancer	Drugs of choice	Some alternative or additional drugs
	Maintenance: Mercapto-purine + methotrexate;	*Maintenance:* Same plus monthly vincristine and prednisone
	High-dose chemotherapy + bone marrow infusion[14]	
Acute myelo-genous leukemia (AML)	*Induction:* Cytarabine + ei-ther daunorubicin or idaru-bicin ± etoposide	High-dose cytarabine + daunorubicin or idarubicin Additional drugs for induc-tion or post induction in-clude: vincristine, cyclo-phosphamide, methotrex-ate, mitoxantrone, fludara-bine, carboplatin, topo-tecan, thioguanine, gem-tuzumab[15]
	For acute promyelocytic leukemia (APL): Tretinoin ± further induction therapy *CNS prophylaxis:* Intrathe-cal cytarabine or metho-trexate ± intrathecal hydro-cortisone *Post Induction:* High-dose cytarabine ± other drugs; High-dose chemotherapy + bone marrow infusion[14]	For acute promyelocytic leukemia: arsenic trioxide
Chronic lympho-cytic leukemia (CLL)	Fludarabine ± cyclophos-phamide; Chlorambucil or cyclophosphamide ± pred-nisone	Cyclophosphamide + vin-cristine + prednisone ± doxorubicin; alemtuzu-mab; cladribine; pentosta-tin High-dose chemotherapy + bone marrow infusion

† Available in the USA for investigational use only.
13. The vitamin A analogue isotretinoin can control pre-neoplastic lesions (leuko-plakia), and decrease the rate of second primary tumors (SE Benner et al, J Natl Cancer Inst 1994; 86:140).
14. Patients with a poor prognosis initially, or those who relapse after remission.
15. Medical Letter 2000; 42:67

Cancer	Drugs of choice	Some alternative or additional drugs
Leukemia *(continued)*		
Chronic myelo-genous leukemia (CML)[16]		
Chronic phase	Interferon alfa ± cytara-bine; High-dose chemotherapy + bone marrow infusion ± donor lymphocyte infu-sions	Imatinib (STI-571)[17]; hy-droxyurea; busulfan; homoharringtonine[†,18]
Accelerated	Cytarabine + daunorubicin or idarubicin; High-dose chemotherapy + bone marrow infusion	Imatinib (STI-571)[17]; hy-droxyurea; busulfan; inter-feron alfa
Blast phase	*Lymphoid:* Vincristine + prednisone + asparaginase + doxorubicin or daunoru-bicin ± cyclophosphamide + intrathecal methotrexate (± maintenance with mer-captopurine + methotrex-ate) *Myeloid:* Cytarabine + dau-norubicin or idarubicin	Imatinib (STI-571)[17]; azaci-tidine[†]; vincristine ± pli-camycin; High dose chemotherapy + bone marrow infusion
Hairy cell leukemia	Cladribine; Pentostatin	Interferon alfa
Liver	Hepatic intra-arterial flox-uridine, cisplatin, doxoru-bicin or mitomycin	Doxorubicin; fluorouracil
Lung		
Non-small cell	Paclitaxel + cisplatin or carboplatin; Cisplatin + vi-norelbine; Gemcitabine + cisplatin	Mitomycin + vinblastine + cisplatin (MVP); mitomycin + ifosfamide with mesna + cisplatin (MIC); docetax-el[19]; irinotecan; cisplatin + etoposide; vinorelbine

16. Allogeneic HLA-identical sibling bone marrow transplantation can cure 30% to 70% of patients with CML in chronic phase, 15% to 25% of patients in accelerated phase and <15% in acute phase. Disease-free survival after bone marrow transplantation is adversely influenced by age >50 years, duration of disease >3 years from diag-nosis, and use of one-antigen-mismatched or matched unrelated donor marrow. In-terferon alfa may be curative in patients with chronic phase CML who achieve a complete cytogenetic response (about 10%). Chemotherapy alone is palliative.

17. Medical Letter 2001; 43:49

Cancer	Drugs of choice	Some alternative or additional drugs
Lung *(continued)*		
Small cell	Cisplatin or carboplatin + etoposide (PE)	Topotecan; cyclophosphamide + doxorubicin + vincristine (CAV); paclitaxel; irinotecan; docetaxel; etoposide + ifosfamide with mesna + cisplatin (VIP); ifosfamide with mesna + carboplatin + etoposide (ICE)
Lymphomas		
Hodgkin's lymphoma[20]	Doxorubicin + bleomycin + vinblastine + dacarbazine (ABVD)	Alternating MOPP (mechlorethamine + vincristine + procarbazine + prednisone)/ABVD; Stanford V Regimen (mechlorethamine + doxorubicin + etoposide + vincristine + vinblastine + bleomycin + prednisone); High-dose chemotherapy + bone marrow or peripheral-blood stem-cell infusion
Non-Hodgkin's lymphomas		
High Grade[21]		
Burkitt's	Cyclophosphamide + doxorubicin + vincristine + prednisone (CHOP) + high dose methotrexate + intrathecal methotrexate; Cyclophosphamide + doxorubicin + vincristine + etoposide + bleomycin + methotrexate + prednisone	High-dose chemotherapy + bone marrow infusion
Lymphoblastic	Cyclophosphamide + doxorubicin + vincristine + prednisone (CHOP) + asparaginase + maintenance with methotrexate + mercaptopurine + intrathecal methotrexate ± cytarabine	High-dose chemotherapy + bone marrow infusion

18. S O'Brien et al, Blood 1999; 93:4149
19. V Georgoulias et al, Lancet 2001; 357:1478

Cancer	Drugs of choice	Some alternative or additional drugs
Non-Hodgkin's lymphomas *(continued)*		
Intermediate Grade[21] Diffuse large-cell, diffuse small-cell, diffuse large-cell and small-cell, follicular large cell	Cyclophosphamide + doxorubicin + vincristine + prednisone (CHOP) ± intrathecal methotrexate or cytarabine	Other combination regimens that may include methotrexate, etoposide, cytarabine, bleomycin, procarbazine, mechlorethamine, dexamethasone, cisplatin, mitoxantrone; High-dose chemotherapy + bone marrow or peripheral-blood stem-cell infusion
Low Grade[22] Follicular small cleaved cell, follicular mixed, small cleaved and large cell	Cyclophosphamide or chlorambucil; Cyclophosphamide + vincristine + prednisone ± doxorubicin; Fludarabine; Rituximab	Cladribine; interferon alfa; etoposide; High-dose chemotherapy + bone marrow or peripheral-blood stem-cell infusion
Cutaneous T-cell	Topical mechlorethamine or carmustine; PUVA (psoralen + ultraviolet A)	Bexarotene[23]; denileukin; isotretinoin; pentostatin; fludarabine; cladribine; methotrexate;
	Systemic chemotherapy as in other non-Hodgkin's lymphomas	Photophoresis (extracorporeal photochemotherapy)
Melanoma	*Adjuvant:* Interferon alfa *Metastatic:* Dacarbazine	Dacarbazine + cisplatin + vinblastine ± interferon alfa + interleukin-2; interferon alfa; interleukin-2

20. Early-stage Hodgkin's disease with no unfavorable features may be treated with radiation alone, or with radiation plus an abbreviated course of chemotherapy (e.g. 4-6 cycles of ABVD).
21. Combined modality therapy with 3 cycles of CHOP chemotherapy followed by involved-field irradiation has been shown to be superior to 8 cyles of CHOP alone in localized intermediate or high-grade NHL (TP Miller et al, N Engl J Med 1998; 339:21).
22. Lymphoma of mucosa-associated lymphoid tissue (MALT) is generally treated similarly to other low-grade lymphomas. When affecting the stomach, however, it is often associated with *Helicobacter pylori* infection, and treatment with omeprazole *(Prilosec)*, amoxicillin *(Amoxil,* and others) and metronidazole *(Flagyl,* and others) alone frequently is sufficient to produce a histologic response.
23. Medical Letter 2000; 42:31

Cancer	Drugs of choice	Some alternative or additional drugs
Multiple Myeloma	Melphalan or cyclophosphamide + prednisone; Vincristine + doxorubicin + dexamethasone (VAD)	Vincristine + carmustine + melphalan + cyclophosphamide + prednisone (VBMCP); etoposide + dexamethasone + cytarabine + cisplatin (EDAP); high-dose dexamethasone; interferon alfa; thalidomide; arsenic trioxide; High-dose chemotherapy + bone marrow or peripheral-blood stem-cell infusion ± donor lymphocyte infusions
Neuroblastoma	Doxorubicin + cyclophosphamide + cisplatin + etoposide or teniposide; High-dose chemotherapy + bone marrow or peripheral-blood stem-cell infusion followed by isotretinoin	Carboplatin; vincristine; topotecan
Osteosarcoma	High-dose methotrexate + doxorubicin + cisplatin	Doxorubicin + cisplatin + methotrexate + ifosfamide with mesna; etoposide + ifosfamide with mesna; ifosfamide with mesna + cisplatin + etoposide (ICE); dactinomycin; vincristine
Ovarian		
Germ Cell Tumor	Bleomycin + etoposide + cisplatin (BEP)	Vincristine + dactinomycin + cisplatin; etoposide + cisplatin or carboplatin
Epithelial	Cisplatin or carboplatin + paclitaxel	Topotecan; cyclophosphamide; ifosfamide with mesna; tamoxifen; melphalan; altretamine; oral etoposide; docetaxel; liposomal doxorubicin; gemcitabine; interferon gamma[24]; oxaliplatin†
Pancreatic	*Adjuvant and localized unresectable*: Fluorouracil *Metastatic*: Gemcitabine	Doxorubicin; mitomycin

24. GH Windbichler et al, Br J Cancer 2000; 82:1138

Cancer	Drugs of choice	Some alternative or additional drugs
Pheochromocytoma	Cyclophosphamide + vincristine + dacarbazine (CVD)	^{131}I-meta-iodobenzyl guanidine (^{131}I MIBG); streptozocin
Prostate	Gonadotropin-releasing hormone (GnRH) agonists (leuprolide or goserelin) ± antiandrogen (flutamide, bicalutamide, or nilutamide)	Mitoxantrone + prednisone; estramustine + docetaxel or vinblastine or paclitaxel; doxorubicin + ketoconazole; ketoconazole + prednisone; megestrol acetate
Renal	Interleukin-2	Interferon alfa
Retinoblastoma	Doxorubicin + cyclophosphamide ± vincristine ± cisplatin ± etoposide; Intrathecal methotrexate ± cytarabine ± hydrocortisone	Carboplatin; ifosfamide with mesna
Rhabdomyosarcoma	Vincristine + dactinomycin + either cyclophosphamide (VAC) or ifosfamide with mesna	Doxorubicin; melphalan; cisplatin; etoposide
Sarcomas, soft tissue (adult)	Ifosfamide with mesna + doxorubicin ± dacarbazine	Doxorubicin + cisplatin + mitomycin; vincristine; cyclophosphamide; epirubicin
Testicular	Cisplatin + etoposide ± bleomycin (PEB)	Ifosfamide with mesna + cisplatin + etoposide or vinblastine; paclitaxel; gemcitabine; High-dose chemotherapy + bone marrow or peripheral-blood stem-cell infusion
Thyroid, anaplastic	Doxorubicin; Cisplatin	
Wilms' tumor	Dactinomycin + vincristine ± doxorubicin ± cyclophosphamide	Ifosfamide with mesna; etoposide; carboplatin or cisplatin; High-dose chemotherapy + bone marrow or peripheral-blood stem-cell infusion

TABLE II — TOXICITY OF SOME ANTICANCER DRUGS

Drug	Acute toxicity*	Delayed toxicity*
Alitretinoin (*Panretin* – Ligand Pharmaceuticals)	Erythema, rash, pruritus	Continued application may result in worsening acute symptoms and also edema and vesiculation
Altretamine (hexamethylmelamine; *Hexalen* – US Bioscience)	Nausea and vomiting	**Bone marrow depression;** CNS depression; peripheral neuropathy; visual hallucinations; ataxia; tremors; alopecia; rash
Alemtuzumab (*Campath* – Berlex)	Fever, rigors, fatigue, musculoskeletal pain, dyspnea, hypotension, urticaria	**Bone marrow depression**
Anastrozole (*Arimidex* – Zeneca)	Nausea; diarrhea; hot flashes; headache	Asthenia; pain (bone pain, back pain); dyspnea; peripheral edema
Arsenic trioxide (*Trisenox* – Cell Therapeutics)	"Retinoic acid syndrome" (fever, dyspnea, pulmonary infiltrates, pleural effusions, peripheral edema, hypotension); fatigue; musculoskeletal pain; prolongation of QT interval and cardiac arrhythmias; hyperglycemia	Peripheral neuropathy; dysesthesias; rash; alopecia; renal toxicity; myelosuppression
Asparaginase (*Elspar* – Merck; *Kidrolase* in Canada)	Nausea and vomiting; fever; chills; headache; hypersensitivity, anaphylaxis; abdominal pain; hyperglycemia leading to coma	CNS depression or hyperexcitability; acute hemorrhagic pancreatitis; coagulation defects; thrombosis; renal damage; hepatic damage
†Azacitidine (ladakamycin; *Mylosar* – Pharmacia)	Nausea and vomiting; diarrhea; fever; rash; drowsiness	**Bone marrow depression;** hepatic damage; muscle pain and weakness; possibly cardiotoxicity
Bexarotene (*Targretin* – Ligand Pharmaceuticals)	Headache, rash	Leukopenia, anemia, asthenia, hypothyroidism, hypertriglyceridemia, hypercholesterolemia, photosensitivity

† Available in the USA for investigational use only.

41

Drug	Acute toxicity*	Delayed toxicity*
BCG (*TheraCys* – Connaught; *Tice BCG* – Organon; *Pacis* – BioChem Pharma)	Bladder irritation; nausea and vomiting; fever; sepsis	Granulomatous pyelonephritis; hepatitis; urethral obstruction; epididymitis; renal abscess
Bicalutamide (*Casodex* – AstraZeneca)	Nausea; diarrhea; hot flashes; hematuria	Gynecomastia; hepatotoxicity
Bleomycin (*Blenoxane* – Bristol-Myers Oncology, and others)	Nausea and vomiting; fever; anaphylaxis and other allergic reactions; phlebitis at injection site	**Pneumonitis and pulmonary fibrosis**; rash and hyperpigmentation; stomatitis; alopecia; Raynaud's phenomenon; cavitating granulomas; hemorrhagic cystitis
Busulfan (*Myleran* – GlaxoSmithKline)	Nausea and vomiting; diarrhea (rare)	**Bone marrow depression; pulmonary infiltrates and fibrosis**; alopecia; gynecomastia; ovarian failure; hyperpermia; azoospermia; leukemia; chromosome aberrations; cataracts; hepatitis; seizures and veno-occlusive disease with high doses; secondary malignancy with prolonged use
Capecitabine (*Xeloda* – Roche)	Nausea; vomiting	**Palmar-plantar erythrodysesthesia**; diarrhea; stomatitis; dermatitis; bone marrow depression; hyperbilirubinemia; ocular irritation and corneal deposits
Carboplatin (*Paraplatin* – Bristol-Myers Oncology)	Nausea and vomiting	**Bone marrow depression**; peripheral neuropathy; hearing loss; transient cortical blindness; hemolytic anemia

* Dose-limiting effects are in bold type. Cutaneous reactions (sometimes severe), hyperpigmentation, and ocular toxicity have been reported with virtually all nonhormonal anticancer drugs. For adverse interactions with other drugs, see *The Medical Letter Handbook of Adverse Drug Interactions*, 2001.

Drug	Acute toxicity*	Delayed toxicity*
Carmustine (BCNU; *BiCNU* – Bristol-Myers Oncology; *Gliadel* – Guilford)	Nausea and vomiting; local phlebitis	**Bone marrow depression (cumulative) with delayed leukopenia and thrombocytopenia** (may be prolonged); pulmonary fibrosis (may be irreversible); delayed renal damage; reversible liver damage; leukemia; myocardial ischemia; veno-occlusive disease of liver after transplantation doses
Chlorambucil (*Leukeran* – GlaxoSmithKline)	Nausea and vomiting	**Bone marrow depression**; pulmonary infiltrates and fibrosis; leukemia; hepatic toxicity; sterility
†Chlorozotocin (*DCNU* – Dome)	Similar to streptozocin, but less nausea and vomiting	Similar to streptozocin, but **leukopenia** and **thrombocytopenia** are common
Cisplatin (Cis-DDP; *Platinol* – Bristol-Myers Oncology)	Nausea and vomiting; diarrhea; hypersensitivity reactions	**Renal damage**; ototoxicity; bone marrow depression; hemolysis; hypomagnesemia; peripheral neuropathy; hypocalcemia; hypokalemia; Raynaud's phenomenon; sterility; hypophosphatemia; hyperuricemia; anorexia
Cladribine (2-chlorodeoxyadenosine; 2-CdA; *Leustatin* – Ortho-Biotech)	Fever	**Bone marrow depression**; immunosuppression; peripheral neuropathy with high doses
Cyclophosphamide (*Cytoxan* – Bristol-Myers Oncology; *Neosar* – Pharmacia)	Nausea and vomiting; Type I (anaphylactoid) hypersensitivity; facial burning and metallic taste with IV administration; visual blurring	**Bone marrow depression**; alopecia; hemorrhagic cystitis; sterility (may be temporary); pulmonary infiltrates and fibrosis; hyponatremia; leukemia; bladder cancer; inappropriate ADH secretion; cardiac toxicity; amenorrhea

Drug	Acute toxicity*	Delayed toxicity*
Cytarabine HCl (*Cytosar-U* – Pharmacia, and others)	Nausea and vomiting; diarrhea; anaphylaxis; sudden respiratory distress with high doses	**Bone marrow depression**; conjunctivitis; megaloblastosis; oral ulceration; hepatic damage; fever; pulmonary edema and central and peripheral neurotoxicity with high doses; rhabdomyolysis; pancreatitis when used with asparaginase; rash
Dacarbazine (*DTIC-Dome* – Bayer)	Nausea and vomiting; diarrhea; anaphylaxis; pain on administration; phlebitis at infusion site	**Bone marrow depression**; alopecia; flu-like syndrome; renal impairment; hepatic necrosis; facial flushing; paresthesia; photosensitivity; urticarial rash
Dactinomycin (*Cosmegen* – Merck)	Nausea and vomiting; hepatic toxicity with ascites; diarrhea; severe local tissue damage and necrosis on extravasation; anaphylactoid reaction	**Stomatitis**; **oral ulceration**; **bone marrow depression**; alopecia; folliculitis; dermatitis in previously irradiated areas
Daunorubicin HCl (*Cerubidine* – Bedford, and others)	Nausea and vomiting; diarrhea; red urine (not hematuria); severe local tissue damage and necrosis on extravasation; transient ECG changes; facial flushing; anaphylactoid reaction	**Bone marrow depression**; **cardiotoxicity** (may be delayed for years); alopecia; stomatitis; anorexia; diarrhea; fever and chills; dermatitis in previously irradiated areas; skin and nail pigmentation; photosensitivity
Liposomal daunorubicin (*DaunoXome* – Gilead)	Less nausea and vomiting; no red urine; less local tissue damage; infusion reactions	Less cardiotoxicity; minimal alopecia
Denileukin diftitox (*Ontak* – Ligand Pharmaceuticals)	Hypersensitivity reactions (hypotension, back pain, dyspnea, rash, chest tightness, tachycardia, dysphagia); chills; fever; headache; nausea and vomiting; diarrhea; pruritus	Vascular leak syndrome (hypotension, edema, hypoalbuminemia); anemia; infection; anorexia; asthenia; increased aminotransferase activity; hypocalcemia

* Dose-limiting effects are in bold type. Cutaneous reactions (sometimes severe), hyperpigmentation, and ocular toxicity have been reported with virtually all nonhormonal anticancer drugs. For adverse interactions with other drugs, see *The Medical Letter Handbook of Adverse Drug Interactions*, 2001.

Drug	Acute toxicity*	Delayed toxicity*
Diethylstilbestrol (*Stilphostrol* – Bayer)	Nausea and vomiting; abdominal cramps; headache	Gynecomastia in males; breast tenderness; loss of libido; thrombophlebitis and thromboembolism; hepatic injury; sodium retention with edema; hypertension; change in menstrual flow
Docetaxel (*Taxotere* – Aventis)	Hypersensitivity reactions; nausea and vomiting	**Bone marrow depression**; peripheral neuropathy; fluid retention (including generalized edema and pleural effusions); myalgia; alopecia; mucositis; cutaneous fibrosis
Doxorubicin HCl (*Adriamycin* – Pharmacia, and others)	Nausea and vomiting; red urine (not hematuria); severe local tissue damage and necrosis on extravasation; diarrhea; fever; transient ECG changes; ventricular arrhythmia; anaphylactoid reaction	**Bone marrow depression**; **cardiotoxicity** (may be delayed for years); alopecia; stomatitis; anorexia; conjunctivitis; acral pigmentation; dermatitis in previously irradiated areas; acral erythrodysesthesia; hyperuricemia; leukemia
Liposomal doxorubicin (*Doxil* – Alza)	Less nausea and vomiting; no red urine; less local tissue damage; infusion reactions	Less cardiotoxicity; minimal alopecia; palmar-plantar and acral dysesthesia
Epirubicin (*Ellence* – Pharmacia; *Pharmorubicin* in Canada)	Local tissue damage; red urine; nausea and vomiting; ECG changes; arrhythmias; anaphylactoid reaction	**Bone marrow depression**; alopecia; paresthesias; fatigue; cardiotoxicity; leukemia
Estramustine phosphate sodium (*Emcyt* – Pharmacia)	Nausea and vomiting; diarrhea	Mild gynecomastia; increased frequency of vascular accidents; myelosuppression (uncommon); edema; dyspnea; pulmonary infiltrates and fibrosis; decreased glucose tolerance; thrombosis; hypertension

Drug	Acute toxicity*	Delayed toxicity*
Etoposide (VP-16; *VePesid* – Bristol-Myers Oncology, and others)	Nausea and vomiting; diarrhea; fever; hypotension; hypersensitivity reactions; phlebitis at infusion site	**Bone marrow depression**; rashes; alopecia; peripheral neuropathy; mucositis and hepatic damage with high doses; leukemia
Exemestane (*Aromasin* – Pharmacia)	Hot flashes, nausea	Peripheral edema and weight gain, fatigue
Floxuridine (*FUDR* – Roche)	Nausea and vomiting; diarrhea	**Oral and gastrointestinal ulceration; bone marrow depression**; alopecia; dermatitis; hepatic dysfunction with hepatic infusion
Fludarabine (*Fludara* – Berlex)	Nausea and vomiting	**Bone marrow depression**; immunosuppression; CNS effects; visual disturbances; renal damage with higher doses; pulmonary infiltrates
Fluorouracil (5-FU; *Adrucil* – Pharmacia, and others)	Nausea and vomiting; diarrhea; mucositis; hypersensitivity reaction (rare)	**Oral and GI ulcers; bone marrow depression**; diarrhea (especially with fluorouracil and leucovorin); neurological defects, usually cerebellar; cardiac arrhythmias; angina pectoris; alopecia; hyperpigmentation; palmarplantar erythrodysesthesia; conjunctivitis; heart failure; seizures
Fluoxymesterone (*Halotestin* – Pharmacia)	Nausea and vomiting	Menstrual changes; gynecomastia; androgenic effects; hepatic toxicity
Flutamide (*Eulexin* – Schering, *Euflex* in Canada)	Nausea; diarrhea; hot flashes	Gynecomastia; hepatic toxicity
Gallium nitrate (*Ganite* – SoloPak)	Hypocalcemia	**Hypophosphatemia**; nephrotoxicity; anemia; optic neuritis

* Dose-limiting effects are in bold type. Cutaneous reactions (sometimes severe), hyperpigmentation, and ocular toxicity have been reported with virtually all nonhormonal anticancer drugs. For adverse interactions with other drugs, see *The Medical Letter Handbook of Adverse Drug Interactions*, 2001.

Drug	Acute toxicity*	Delayed toxicity*
Gemcitabine (*Gemzar* – Lilly)	Fatigue; nausea and vomiting	Bone marrow depression, especially thrombocytopenia; edema; pulmonary toxicity; anal pruritus
Gemtuzumab (*Mylotarg* – Wyeth-Ayerst)	Fever; chills; nausea; hypotension	Bone marrow depression; increased aminotransferase activity
Goserelin (*Zoladex* – AstraZeneca)	Transient increase in bone pain; transient increase in tumor mass, resulting in ureteral obstruction and/or spinal cord compression in patients with metastatic prostate cancer; hot flashes	Impotence; testicular atrophy; gynecomastia; allergic reactions
†Homoharringtonine (HHT-Oncopharm)	Hypotension; tachycardia and arrhythmias; headache; nausea and vomiting; diarrhea; hyperglycemia; fluid retention; myalgias	**Bone marrow depression**; fatigue; elevated transaminase levels
Hydroxyurea (*Hydrea* – Bristol-Myers Oncology, and others)	Nausea and vomiting; allergic reactions to tartazine dye	**Bone marrow depression**; stomatitis; dysuria; alopecia; rare neurological disturbances; pulmonary infiltrates
Idarubicin (*Idamycin* – Pharmacia)	Nausea and vomiting; tissue damage on extravasation	**Bone marrow depression**; alopecia; stomatitis; myocardial toxicity; diarrhea
Ifosfamide (*Ifex* – Bristol-Myers Oncology)	Nausea and vomiting; confusion; nephrotoxicity; metabolic acidosis and renal Fanconi's syndrome; **cardiac toxicity** with high doses	**Bone marrow depression**; **hemorrhagic cystitis** (prevented by concurrent mesna); alopecia; inappropriate ADH secretion; renal failure; neurotoxicity (somnolence, hallucinations, blurring of vision, coma)
Imatinib (STI-571; *Gleevec* – Novartis)	Nausea and vomiting; rash; diarrhea; muscle cramps; increased aminotransferase activity	**Bone marrow depression**; pulmonary, periorbital and pedal edema

Drug	Acute toxicity*	Delayed toxicity*
Interferon alfa-2a, alfa-2b, alfa-n3 (*Roferon-A* – Roche, *Intron A* – Schering, *Alferon-N* – Interferon)	Fever; chills; myalgias; fatigue; nausea; diarrhea; headache; arthralgias; hypotension	Bone marrow depression; anorexia; neutropenia; anemia; confusion; depression; renal toxicity; possible hepatic injury; facial and peripheral edema; cardiac arrhythmias; rhabdomyolysis
Interleukin-2 (aldesleukin; *Proleukin* – Chiron)	**Fever; fluid retention; hypotension; respiratory distress;** rash; anemia; thrombocytopenia; nausea and vomiting; diarrhea; capillary leak syndrome; nephrotoxicity; myocardial toxicity; hepatotoxicity; erythema nodosum; neutrophil chemotactic defects	Neuropsychiatric disorders; hypothyroidism; nephrotic syndrome; possibly acute leukoencephalopathy; brachial plexopathy; bowel perforation
Irinotecan (*Camptosar* – Pharmacia)	Nausea and vomiting; **early diarrhea (<24 hours);** fever	**Late diarrhea** (>24 hours); **mucositis; bone marrow depression;** anorexia; asthenia; alopecia; abdominal cramping and pain
Isotretinoin (*Accutane* – Roche)	Fatigue; headache; nausea and vomiting; pruritus	**Teratogenicity;** cheilitis; xerostomia; rash; conjunctivitis and eye irritation; bone and joint pain; anorexia; hypertriglyceridemia; pseudotumor cerebri
Letrozole (*Femara* – Novartis)	Hot flashes; nausea and vomiting; headache	Peripheral edema and weight gain; dyspnea; fatigue; musculoskeletal pain; arthralgia; constipation; diarrhea; rare thromboembolic events
Leucovorin (*Wellcovorin* – GlaxoSmithKline, and others)	Hypersensitivity reactions; nausea, diarrhea	

* Dose-limiting effects are in bold type. Cutaneous reactions (sometimes severe), hyperpigmentation, and ocular toxicity have been reported with virtually all nonhormonal anticancer drugs. For adverse interactions with other drugs, see *The Medical Letter Handbook of Adverse Drug Interactions*, 2001.

Drug	Acute toxicity*	Delayed toxicity*
Leuprolide acetate (*Lupron, Lupron Depot* – TAP, and others)	Transient increase in bone pain; transient increase in tumor mass, resulting in ureteral obstruction and/or spinal cord compression in patients with metastatic prostate cancer; hot flashes; hematuria	Impotence; testicular atrophy; CNS effects; gynecomastia; peripheral edema; allergic reactions
Lomustine (CCNU; *CeeNU* – Bristol-Myers Oncology)	Nausea and vomiting	**Bone marrow depression** (cumulative) with delayed leukopenia and thrombocytopenia (may be prolonged); transient elevation of transaminase activity; neurological reactions; pulmonary fibrosis; renal damage; leukemia
Mechlorethamine HCl (nitrogen mustard; *Mustargen* – Merck)	Nausea and vomiting; local reaction and phlebitis	**Bone marrow depression**; alopecia; diarrhea; oral ulcers; leukemia; amenorrhea; sterility; hyperuricemia
Megestrol acetate (*Megace* – Bristol-Myers Oncology, and others)	Nausea and vomiting; headache	Menstrual changes; hot flashes; thrombophlebitis and thromboembolism; fluid retention; edema; weight gain
Melphalan (*Alkeran* – GlaxoSmithKline)	Mild nausea; hypersensitivity reactions	**Bone marrow depression** (especially platelets); pulmonary infiltrates and fibrosis; amenorrhea; sterility; leukemia
Mercaptopurine (*Purinethol* – GlaxoSmithKline)	Nausea and vomiting; diarrhea	**Bone marrow depression**; cholestasis and rarely hepatic necrosis; oral and intestinal ulcers; pancreatitis
Mesna (*Mesnex* – Bristol-Myers Oncology; *Uromitexan* in Canada)	Nausea and vomiting; diarrhea; allergic reactions	

Drug	Acute toxicity*	Delayed toxicity*
Methotrexate (MTX; *Folex* – Pharmacia, and others)	Nausea and vomiting; diarrhea; fever; hepatic necrosis; hypersensitivity reactions	**Oral and gastrointestinal ulceration**, perforation may occur; **bone marrow depression**; hepatic toxicity including cirrhosis; renal toxicity; **pulmonary infiltrates and fibrosis**; osteoporosis; conjunctivitis; alopecia; depigmentation; menstrual dysfunction; encephalopathy; infertility; lymphoma
Mitomycin (*Mutamycin* – Bristol-Myers Oncology, and others)	Nausea and vomiting; tissue necrosis; fever	**Bone marrow depression** (cumulative) with delayed leukopenia and thrombocytopenia; stomatitis; alopecia; acute pulmonary toxicity; pulmonary fibrosis; cardiotoxicity; hepatotoxicity; renal toxicity; amenorrhea; hemolytic-uremic syndrome; bladder calcification (with intravesical administration)
Mitotane (o,p'-DDD; *Lysodren* – Bristol-Myers Oncology)	Nausea and vomiting; diarrhea	**CNS depression**; rash; visual disturbances; adrenal insufficiency; hematuria; hemorrhagic cystitis; albuminuria; hypertension; orthostatic hypotension; cataracts; prolonged bleeding time
Mitoxantrone HCl (*Novantrone* – Immunex)	Blue-green pigment in urine; blue-green sclera; nausea and vomiting; fever; phlebitis	**Bone marrow depression**; cardiotoxicity; alopecia; white hair; skin lesions; hepatic damage; renal failure; extravasation necrosis; stomatitis
Nilutamide (*Nilandron* – Aventis)	Nausea and vomiting; hot flashes; alcohol intolerance	Delayed adaptation to darkness; hepatic toxicity; gynecomastia; interstitial pneumonitis

* Dose-limiting effects are in bold type. Cutaneous reactions (sometimes severe), hyperpigmentation, and ocular toxicity have been reported with virtually all nonhormonal anticancer drugs. For adverse interactions with other drugs, see *The Medical Letter Handbook of Adverse Drug Interactions*, 2001.

Drug	Acute toxicity*	Delayed toxicity*
Octreotide (*Sandostatin* – Novartis)	Nausea and vomiting; diarrhea	Steatorrhea; gallstones
†Oxaliplatin (*Eloxatine* – Sanofi-Synthelabo Research)	Pharyngolaryngeal dysesthesias; paresthesias; nausea and vomiting; rare cases of anaphylaxis (reduced systolic blood pressure, flushing, tachycardia, respiratory distress)	Peripheral neuropathy; bone marrow depression; diarrhea
Paclitaxel (*Taxol* – Bristol-Myers Oncology)	Hypersensitivity reactions	**Bone marrow depression;** peripheral neuropathy; alopecia; arthralgias; myalgias; cardiac toxicity; mucositis
Pegaspargase (PEG-L-asparaginase; *Oncaspar* – Aventis)	Similar to asparaginase	Similar to asparaginase
Pentostatin (2'-deoxycoformycin; *Nipent* – SuperGen)	Nausea and vomiting; rash	Nephrotoxicity; CNS depression; **bone marrow depression;** respiratory failure; hepatic toxicity; arthralgia; myalgia; photophobia; conjunctivitis
Plicamycin (*Mithricin* – Pfizer)	Nausea and vomiting; soft tissue damage with extravasation	Bone marrow depression, especially **thrombocytopenia;** coagulopathy and hemorrhage; renal damage; hepatic toxicity
Procarbazine HCl (*Matulane* – Roche, *Natulan* in Canada)	Nausea and vomiting; CNS depression; disulfiram-like effect with alcohol; adverse interactions typical of a monoamine oxidase (MAO) inhibitor	**Bone marrow depression;** stomatitis; peripheral neuropathy; pneumonitis; leukemia
Rituximab (*Rituxan* – IDEC Pharmaceutical/Genentech)	Fever; chills; nausea; vomiting; headache; myalgia; pruritus; rash; pain at sites of disease; severe hypersensitivity reactions (hypotension, bronchospasm, angioedema); cardiac arrhythmias; renal failure	Bone marrow depression; mucocutaneous reactions including Stevens-Johnson syndrome and toxic epidermal necrolysis

Drug	Acute toxicity*	Delayed toxicity*
Streptozocin (*Zanosar* – Pharmacia)	Nausea and vomiting; local pain	**Renal damage**; hypoglycemia; hyperglycemia; liver damage; diarrhea; bone marrow depression (uncommon); fever; eosinophilia; nephrogenic diabetes insipidus
Tamoxifen citrate (*Nolvadex* – AstraZeneca; *Tamofen* in Canada)	Hot flashes; nausea and vomiting; transient increased bone or tumor pain	Vaginal bleeding and discharge; hypercalcemia; rash; thrombocytopenia; peripheral edema; depression; dizziness; headache; decreased visual acuity; cataracts; purpuric vasculitis; thromboembolism; endometrial cancer
Temozolomide (*Temodar* – Schering)	Nausea and vomiting; headache	Bone marrow depression, especially thrombocytopenia and neutropenia; asthenia; fatigue
Teniposide (*Vumon* – Bristol-Myers Oncology)	Severe hypersensitivity reactions; nausea and vomiting; diarrhea; phlebitis at infusion site	**Bone marrow depression**; alopecia; mucositis; rash; hepatic toxicity; leukemia
Thalidomide (*Thalomid* – Celgene)	Rash; pruritus; headache; dizziness; drowsiness; somnolence; constipation; rarely toxic epidermal necrolysis	Severe birth defects; peripheral neuropathy; neutropenia
Thioguanine (GlaxoSmithKline; *Lanvis* in Canada)	Occasional nausea and vomiting; diarrhea	**Bone marrow depression**; hepatic damage; stomatitis
Thiotepa (*Thioplex* – Immunex)	Nausea and vomiting; rare hypersensitivity reaction	**Bone marrow depression**; menstrual dysfunction; interference with spermatogenesis; leukemia; mucositis with high doses
Topotecan (*Hycamtin* – GlaxoSmithKline)	Nausea and vomiting; diarrhea; headache; flu-like symptoms	**Bone marrow depression**; asthenia; stomatitis; alopecia; abdominal pain

Drug	Acute toxicity*	Delayed toxicity*
Toremifene (*Fareston* – Schering)	Hot flashes; nausea and vomiting	Vaginal bleeding and discharge; peripheral edema; dizziness; increased aminotransferase activity; hypercalcemia; rare thromboembolic events
Trastuzumab (*Herceptin* – Genentech)	Fever; chills; rigors; nausea and vomiting; headache; rash; hypotension; hypersensitivity reactions (hypotension, angioedema, tachycardia, respiratory distress)	Cardiac dysfunction, including congestive heart failure, particularly when combined with an anthracycline; diarrhea
Tretinoin (*Vesanoid* – Roche)	**Headache; xerosis;** pruritus; "retinoic acid syndrome" (fever, dyspnea, pulmonary infiltrates, pleural effusions, peripheral edema, hypotension); arthralgias; myalgias	**Cheilitis; teratogenicity;** rashes; leucocytosis; hypertriglyceridemia; pseudotumor cerebri; thrombophlebitis
Valrubicin (*Valstar* – Medeva)	Bladder irritation	
Vinblastine sulfate (*Velban* – Lilly, and others; *Velbe* in Canada)	Nausea and vomiting; local reaction and tissue damage with extravasation	**Bone marrow depression;** alopecia; peripheral neuropathy; stomatitis; jaw pain; muscle pain; paralytic ileus
Vincristine sulfate (*Oncovin* – Lilly, and others)	Tissue damage with extravasation	**Peripheral neuropathy;** alopecia; mild bone marrow depression; constipation; paralytic ileus; jaw pain; inappropriate ADH secretion; optic atrophy
Vinorelbine tartrate (*Navelbine* – GlaxoSmithKline)	Nausea and vomiting; injection site reactions (erythema, discoloration, phlebitis, pain)	**Bone marrow depression;** alopecia; anorexia; stomatitis; asthenia; peripheral neuropathy; constipation

* Dose-limiting effects are in bold type. Cutaneous reactions (sometimes severe), hyperpigmentation, and ocular toxicity have been reported with virtually all nonhormonal anticancer drugs. For adverse interactions with other drugs, see *The Medical Letter Handbook of Adverse Drug Interactions*, 2001.

PARTIAL LIST OF BRAND NAMES

Accutane – isotretinoin
*Adriamycin – doxorubicin
*Adrucil – fluorouracil
Alferon N – interferon alfa-n3
Alkeran – melphalan
Arimidex – anastrozole
Aromasin – exemestane
BiCNU – carmustine
*Blenoxane – bleomycin
Campath – alemtuzumab
Camptosar – irinotecan
Casodex – bicalutamide
CeeNU – lomustine
*Cerubidine – daunorubicin
Cosmegen – dactinomycin
Cytadren – aminoglutethimide
*Cytosar-U – cytarabine
*Cytoxan – cyclophosphamide
DaunoXome – liposomal daunorubicin
†DCNU – chlorozotocin
Depo-Provera – medroxyprogesterone acetate
Doxil – liposomal doxorubicin
*DTIC-Dome – dacarbazine
Ellence – epirubicin
†Eloxatine – oxaliplatin
Elspar – asparaginase
Emcyt – estramustine phosphate sodium
Eulexin – flutamide
Fareston – toremifene
Femara – letrozole
Fludara – fludarabine
FUDR – floxuridine
Ganite – gallium nitrate
Gemzar – gemcitabine
Gleevec – imatinib
Gliadel – carmustine wafer
Halotestin – fluoxymesterone
Herceptin – trastuzumab
Hexalen – altretamine
Hycamtin – topotecan

*Hydrea – hydroxyurea
Idamycin – idarubicin
Ifex – ifosfamide
Intron-A – interferon alfa-2b
Kidrolase – asparaginase
Leukeran – chlorambucil
Leustatin – cladribine
*Lupron – leuprolide acetate
Lysodren – mitotane
Matulane – procarbazine
*Megace – megestrol acetate
Mesnex – mesna
Mustargen – mechlorethamine
*Mutamycin – mitomycin
Myleran – busulfan
†Mylosar – azacitidine
Mylotarg – gemtuzumab
Natulan – procarbazine
Navelbine – vinorelbine tartrate
*Neosar – cyclophosphamide
Nilandron – nilutamide
Nipent – pentostatin
Nolvadex – tamoxifen citrate
Novantrone – mitoxantrone
Oncaspar – pegaspargase
*Oncovin – vincristine sulfate
Ontak – denileukin diftitox
Pacis – live BCG
Panretin – alitretinoin
Paraplatin – carboplatin
Pharmorubicin – epirubicin
Platinol – cisplatin
Proleukin – interleukin-2 (aldesleukin)
*Provera – medroxyprogesterone acetate
Purinethol – mercaptopurine
Rituxan – rituximab
Roferon-A – interferon alfa-2a
*Rubex – doxorubicin
Sandostatin – octreotide
Stilphostrol – diethylstilbestrol
Tamofen – tamoxifen

* Also available generically
† Available in the USA for investigational use only.

Tarabine – cytarabine
Targretin – bexarotene
Taxol – paclitaxel
Taxotere – docetaxel
Tegison – etretinate
Temodar – temozolomide
Thalidomid – Thalidomide
TheraCys – live BCG
Thioplex – thiotepa
TiceBCG – live BCG
Trisenox – arsenic thioxide
†*UFT* – tegafur/uracil

Uromitexan – mesna
Valstar – valrubicin
Velban – vinblastine
Velbe – vinblastine
VePesid – etoposide
Vesanoid – tretinoin
Vincasar – vincristine
Vumon – teniposide
Wellcovorin – leucovorin
Xeloda – capecitabine
Zanosar – streptozocin
Zoladex – goserelin

---

* Also available generically
† Available in the USA for investigational use only.

DRUGS FOR CARDIAC ARRHYTHMIAS

The drugs of choice for treatment of common cardiac arrhythmias are listed below. Some drugs are recommended for indications for which they have not been approved by the US Food and Drug Administration. The dosages, adverse effects and therapeutic serum concentrations of each drug are listed in the table that begins on page 64. Antiarrhythmic drugs may themselves cause arrhythmias, which can be fatal. Some of these drugs may increase rather than decrease mortality, especially in patients with structural heart disease.

DRUGS OF CHOICE FOR COMMON ARRHYTHMIAS

Arrhythmia	Drug of choice	Alternatives	Remarks
Atrial fibrillation or flutter[1,2]			
Acute management	Rate control: IV verapamil, diltiazem, a beta-blocker or digoxin		
	Conversion: cardioversion[2]	IV procainamide or ibutilide; single large oral dose of propafenone or flecainide	Ibutilide infusion may increase the effectiveness of DC cardioversion[3]
Chronic treatment	Rate control: oral verapamil, diltiazem, a beta-blocker or digoxin		Radiofrequency ablation of the AV node and pacemaker in highly selected patients

1. Treatment recently reviewed in RH Falk, N Engl J Med 2001; 344:1067.
2. Anticoagulation may be required. Digoxin, verapamil, diltiazem and possibly beta-blockers may be dangerous for patients with Wolff-Parkinson-White syndrome. Patients with Wolff-Parkinson-White syndrome and atrial fibrillation should be treated with IV procainamide or IV amiodarone if hemodynamically stable and, if not, with DC cardioversion.
3. H Oral et al, N Engl J Med 1999; 340:1849.

Arrhythmia	Drug of choice	Alternatives	Remarks
Chronic treatment *(continued)*			
	Maintenance of sinus rhythm[4]: Amiodarone, sotalol, dofetilide, quinidine, procainamide, disopyramide, flecainide or propafenone		Radiofrequency ablation in patients with atrial flutter and in selected cases of atrial fibrillation
Other supraventricular tachycardias[5]	Adenosine, verapamil or diltiazem for termination[6,7]	Esmolol, another beta-blocker or digoxin for termination[6]	DC cardioversion or atrial pacing may be effective for some patients, but are only rarely required. Radiofrequency ablation can cure most patients. Beta-blockers, verapamil, diltiazem, flecainide, propafenone, quinidine, procainamide, disopyramide, amiodarone, sotalol or digoxin may be effective for long-term suppression.

4. Choice of drugs varies with the clinical setting (EN Prystowsky, Am J Cardiol 1998; 82 suppl 4A:3I). The incidence of atrial fibrillation following cardiac surgery can be reduced by preoperative sotalol (JA Gomes et al, J Am Coll Cardiol 1999; 34:334) or beta blockers.

5. These are mostly AV nodal reentry and AV reentry utilizing an accessory atrioventricular connection (bypass tract). Vagotonic maneuvers (such as carotid sinus massage, gagging, or the Valsalva maneuver) that impair AV nodal conduction may be tried first. For rarer forms of supraventricular tachycardia (e.g. atrial tachycardia), drugs are often less effective for suppression; AV nodal blockers (such as digoxin, beta-blockers or calcium-channel blockers) can be used to slow the rate. Radiofrequency ablation can also be used.

6. Digoxin, verapamil, diltiazem and possibly beta-blockers may be dangerous for patients with Wolff-Parkinson-White syndrome.

7. Verapamil and diltiazem should be used with caution in patients receiving intravenous beta-blockers, those with congestive heart failure and those taking oral quinidine.

Arrhythmia	Drug of choice	Alternatives	Remarks
Premature ventricular complexes (PVCs) or non-sustained ventricular tachycardia	No drug therapy indicated for asymptomatic patients without structural heart disease[8]	For symptomatic patients, a beta-blocker	There is no evidence that prolonged suppression with drugs improves survival. For post-MI patients, treatment with a beta-blocker has decreased mortality, and treatment with flecainide or moricizine has increased it.
Sustained ventricular tachycardia[9,10]	Amiodarone for acute treatment[9,10]	Procainamide, lidocaine[9,10]	Long-term therapy[11]: Implantable cardioverter-defibrillator (ICD) Amiodarone
Ventricular fibrillation[12]	Amiodarone[12]	Procainamide[12]	Long-term therapy[11]: Implantable cardioverter-defibrillator (ICD) Amiodarone
Cardiac glycoside-induced ventricular tachyarrhythmias[10,13]	Digoxin-immune Fab (digoxin antibody fragments – Digibind)	Lidocaine, phenytoin	Self-limited if digoxin is stopped. Phenytoin can also be effective. Avoid DC cardioversion and bretylium, except for ventricular fibrillation or sustained ventricular tachycardia. A beta-blocker or procainamide can make heart block worse.

8. One study in asymptomatic patients with non-sustained ventricular tachycardia, coronary disease, reduced ejection fraction and ventricular tachycardia inducible by programmed electrical stimulation reported that treatment with an implantable cardioverter-defibrillator (ICD), but not antiarrhythmics, reduced mortality (AE Buxton et al, N Engl J Med 2000; 341:1882).

9. DC cardioversion is the safest and most effective treatment. It is preferred by most cardiologists for sustained ventricular tachycardia causing hemodynamic compromise.

10. Some ventricular tachycardias can be caused or exacerbated by bradycardia or heart block. In the presence of high-grade heart block, antiarrhythmic drugs can cause cardiac standstill. When high-grade heart block is present, therefore, a temporary pacemaker should be inserted before using antiarrhythmic drugs; pacing may abolish the arrhythmia. When a drug must be used in the presence of heart block, lidocaine is least likely to increase the block.

11. Beta-blockers are often added. If ICD shocks are frequent, antiarrhythmic drugs (sotalol, amiodarone, mexiletine) are often added empirically and if shocks recur, radiofrequency catheter ablation is used.

12. Defibrillation is the treatment of choice; drugs are for prevention of recurrence.

Arrhythmia	Drug of choice	Alternatives	Remarks
Drug-induced Torsades de pointes	IV magnesium sulfate	Cardiac pacing, isoproterenol	Causative agents (e.g., quinidine) should be discontinued. Magnesium sulfate may be effective even in absence of hypomagnesemia. Potassium should be used to raise serum K to between 4.5 and 5.0 mEq/L[13]

13. KCl can be given carefully, 10-20 mEq/hr IV, to patients with low or normal serum potassium concentrations. Extreme care must be taken to keep serum potassium below 5.0 mEq/L. In the presence of heart block not associated with atrial tachycardia, potassium should be withheld if the serum concentration is greater than 4.5 mEq/L because high serum potassium may increase atrioventricular block.

CLASSIFICATION OF ANTIARRHYTHMIC DRUGS — Several approaches have been proposed to classify drugs used for treatment of cardiac arrhythmias. These classifications are based on the premise that drugs with similar electrophysiologic effects are also similar in their therapeutic effects and cardiac toxicity. Agents that appear to be similar in the laboratory may, however, have many different effects in patients. In practice, the choice of drugs is based mainly on controlled trials and clinical experience, especially with cardiac and noncardiac toxicity.

BETA-ADRENERGIC BLOCKERS — Beta-blockers can control the ventricular rate in atrial fibrillation or flutter and terminate paroxysmal supraventricular tachycardias. They are also safer, although somewhat less effective, than other drugs for suppression of symptomatic premature ventricular complexes (PVCs). Sudden withdrawal of a beta-blocker in a patient with angina pectoris can precipitate myocardial ischemia or a cardiac arrhythmia. Drugs in this class approved by the US Food and Drug Administration for treatment of various arrhythmias include **propranolol** (*Inderal*, and others), **acebutolol** (*Sectral*, and others) and **esmolol** (*Brevibloc*). Esmolol is an intravenous cardioselective agent with an elimination half-life of about nine minutes; it is effective in controlling the ventricular response in atrial flutter or fibrillation, particularly after cardiac surgery, and both therapeutic and adverse effects (hypotension, bradycardia) usually disappear within 30 minutes after stopping an infusion. Beta-blockers, except those with intrinsic sympathomimetic activity, decrease both short- and long-term mortality after myocardial infarction, and in patients with heart failure. Other antiarrhythmic drugs (sotalol, amiodarone, propafenone) exert anti-adrenergic actions that likely contribute to their efficacy in some patients.

CALCIUM-CHANNEL BLOCKERS — **Verapamil** (*Calan*, and others) and **diltiazem** (*Cardizem*, and others) prolong AV nodal refractoriness and are effective in terminating many supraventricular tachycardias and slowing the ventricular rate in atrial fibrillation or flutter. Their intravenous use can be complicated by hypotension or bradycardia, especially with concurrent use of other cardiodepressant drugs, in patients with underlying heart disease, and in those with sustained ventricular tachycardia, in whom these drugs can be dangerous (DS Cannom and EN Prystowsky, JAMA 1999; 281:172). Verapamil is also approved for oral use in treating supraventricular arrhythmias. Either diltiazem or verapamil can raise serum digoxin levels, and both interact with many other drugs, including beta-blockers (*The Medical Letter Handbook of Adverse Drug Interactions*, 2001, pages 260 and 440). Usual doses of dihydropyridine calcium-channel blockers—all those available in the USA except for verapamil, diltiazem and bepridil *(Vascor)*—have no antiarrhythmic activity. Bepridil is indicated only for refractory angina; it can cause torsades de pointes.

AMIODARONE AND SOTALOL — Controlled clinical trials in patients with a history of sustained ventricular tachycardia or ventricular fibrillation suggest that these drugs are more effective than older agents such as quinidine or procainamide (The Cascade Investigators, Am J Cardiol 1993; 72:280; JW Mason, N Engl J Med 1993; 329:452). Both drugs, especially amiodarone, have become drugs of choice for these serious arrhythmias.

Orally-administered **amiodarone** (*Cordarone*, and others) can suppress PVCs and nonsustained ventricular tachycardia and prevent recurrences of sustained ventricular tachycardia or fibrillation. In one study amiodarone significantly reduced recurrences of symptomatic atrial fibrillation compared to sotalol or propafenone, even though more patients discontinued amiodarone because of adverse effects (D Roy et al, N Engl J Med 2000; 342:913). Two large trials evaluating use of amiodarone in post-myocardial-infarction patients found no effect on total mortality but a 35% decrease in the incidence of sudden death (DG Julian et al, Lancet 1997; 349:667; JA Cairns et al, Lancet 1997; 349:675). Low doses of the drug have been reported to improve contractility in patients with heart failure; whether the drug decreases mortality in such patients is controversial (HC Doval et al, Lancet 1994; 344:493; SN Singh et al, N Engl J Med 1995; 333:77). Severe adverse effects, including pulmonary toxicity, can occur with usual doses of amiodarone and may be lethal or irreversible or persist for months after treatment is stopped. Increased hepatic enzyme activity is common; cirrhosis and fatal hepatic necrosis have been reported. Thyroid dysfunction is also common (KJ Harjai and AA Licata, Ann Intern Med 1997; 126:63). Low doses of amiodarone appear to cause fewer adverse effects, but blue-gray skin discoloration is common, and rarely optic neuritis can occur and has led to loss of vision (VR Vorperian et al, J Am Coll Cardiol 1997; 30:791).

Intravenous (IV) amiodarone appears to be effective for treatment of ventricular fibrillation (prevention of recurrences) or recurrent, hemodynamically destabilizing ventricular tachycardia, and may be more effective than intravenous bretylium for these indications. In patients with out-of-hospital cardiac arrest, a randomized trial showed improved survival to hospital admission with intravenous amiodarone compared to standard therapy (PJ Kudenchuk et al, N Engl J Med 1999; 341:871). Therefore amiodarone has supplanted lidocaine as the drug of choice in many cardiac arrest situations (Guidelines, Circulation 2000; 102 suppl I:I86). Phlebitis, hypotension, bradyarrhythmias and exacerbation of heart failure are the major adverse effects of IV amiodarone. Although amiodarone prolongs the QT interval, the long-QT-associated ventricular arrhythmia torsades de pointes occurs only rarely with intravenous or oral use of the drug (Medical Letter 1995; 37:114). IV amiodarone is not acutely effective in converting atrial fibrillation to sinus rhythm (E Galve et al, J Am Coll Cardiol 1996; 27:1079; MN Sharif and DG Wyse et al, Can J Cardiol 1998; 14:1241), but can slow ventricular response (G Cotter et al, Eur Heart J 1999; 20:1833). IV followed by oral amiodarone has been reported to be effective in termination of persistant atrial fibrillation (GE Kochia-dakis et al, Am J Cardiol 1999; 83:58).

Amiodarone can increase the serum concentrations, phar-macological effects and toxicity of digoxin, diltiazem, quinidine, procainamide, flecainide, beta-blockers, warfarin and other drugs (*The Medical Letter Handbook of Adverse Drug Interactions*, 2001, page 33).

Sotalol (*Betapace, Betapace AF*, and others) is a non-selective beta-blocker that also prolongs the QT interval. Randomized trials suggest that its effectiveness is equivalent to that of quinidine for prevention of recurrences of atrial fibrillation (JL Anderson and EN Prystowsky, Am Heart J 1999; 137:388). In patients with implant-able cardioverter-defibrillators, use of sotalol reduced the risk of death from any cause or delivery of a first shock for any reason (A Pacifico et al, N Engl J Med 1999; 340:1855). Major adverse effects are those related to beta-blockade and prolongation of the QT inter-val, with a risk of torsades de pointes. Hypokalemia, hypomagne-semia, bradycadia and high drug doses (except quinidine) increase the risk of torsades de pointes with all QT-prolonging drugs.

Dofetilide *(Tikosyn)* is a selective blocker of one specific cardi-ac repolarizing current and has no other pharmacologic effects (JP Mounsey and JP DiMarco, Circulation 2000; 102:2665). It is used orally to convert atrial fibrillation and to maintain sinus rhythm after cardioversion. Placebo-controlled trials have not shown efficacy in ventricular arrhythmias or paroxysmal atrial fibrillation. In patients with advanced heart failure or recent MI, dofetilide de-creased the incidence of rehospitalization for heart failure, possibly by suppressing atrial fibrillation, and did not increase mortality (C Torp-Pedersen et al, N Engl J Med 1999; 341:857). The major risk is torsades de pointes, which occurred in 0.5% to 3.3% of patients in controlled trials. The drug must be started in the hospital and closely monitored. Because of its pharmacologic selectivity, other adverse effects are uncommon.

QUINIDINE, PROCAINAMIDE, DISOPYRAMIDE — Quinidine has largely been supplanted as the drug of choice for oral therapy of many arrhythmias. It is occasionally used in patients with atrial fibrillation or frequent ICD shocks. When quinidine, procainamide or disopyramide are given to a patient with atrial flutter, the ventricular rate may increase as the atrial rate slows; an AV-nodal blocking agent such as digoxin, verapamil or a beta-blocker is usually given first. Quinidine can, however, increase digoxin concentrations to potentially toxic levels, and it also interacts with many other drugs (*The Medical Letter Handbook of Adverse Drug Interactions*, 2001, page 400). Torsades de pointes is the likely cause of "quinidine syncope."

Procainamide (*Pronestyl*, and others) can be given IV more safely than quinidine, although hypotension can occur with high or rapid loading doses. With long-term use, adverse extracardiac effects, such as fever or rash, are fairly common. Many patients develop antinuclear antibodies (ANA) after three to six months of therapy, and up to 30% develop a lupus-like syndrome, which usually disappears slowly when the drug is discontinued. Agranulocytosis unrelated to the lupus reaction occurs in 0.5% of patients. Torsades de pointes has been reported with high concentrations either of the drug or its active metabolite. It should not be used in patients with renal failure.

Disopyramide (*Norpace*, and others) can aggravate heart failure, and anticholinergic effects are often prominent; urinary retention frequently requires discontinuation of the drug. Nevertheless, in some patients it may be tolerated better than quinidine. Torsades de pointes has been reported.

(Text continues on page 70)

DOSAGE AND ADVERSE EFFECTS OF SOME ANTIARRHYTHMIC DRUGS

Drug	Usual dosage* and interval	Effect on ECG
BETA-ADRENERGIC BLOCKERS		
Propranolol (*Inderal*, and others)	PO: 10-80 mg q6h (long-acting formulation available) IV: 1-5 mg total (1 mg/min)	Prolongs PR (±) No Change QRS Bradycardia
Acebutolol (*Sectral*, and others)	PO: 200 mg bid, increase gradually to 600-1200 mg/day	Bradycardia
Esmolol (*Brevibloc*)	IV Loading: 500 µg/kg over one minute, followed by 50 µg/kg/min; titrate to desired effect Usual maintenance: 100 µg/kg/min; maximum 300 µg/kg/min	Sinus bradycardia
CALCIUM-CHANNEL BLOCKERS		
Verapamil HCl (*Calan*, and others)	IV Initial dose: 5-10 mg over 2-3 min; repeat in 15-30 min, if necessary IV Infusion: Initial dose is followed by 0.375 mg/min for 30 min IV Maintenance: 0.125 mg/min PO: 40-120 mg tid or qid (long-acting formulation available)	Prolongs PR Sinus bradycardia
Diltiazem (*Cardizem*, and others)	IV Initial dose: 0.15-0.35 mg/kg (10-25 mg) over 2 min, may be repeated in 15 min IV infusion: 5-15 mg/hr	Prolongs PR Sinus bradycardia
AMIODARONE AND SOTALOL		
Amiodarone (*Cordarone*, and others)	PO Loading: 800-1200 mg/day for 1-2 weeks then 600-800 mg/day for 4 weeks PO Maintenance: 100-400 mg/day IV loading: 150 mg over 10 minutes, which can be repeated once if needed, followed by 360 mg over 6 hours IV Maintenance: 0.25-0.5 mg/min	Prolongs PR, QRS and QT Sinus bradycardia

* Patients with decreased hepatic or renal function may require lower dosage.

† Range of usually effective and tolerated concentrations

Adverse effects	Serum concentrations[†]
Heart block, hypotension, heart failure, bronchospasm, depression	Not used
Hypotension, bradycardia, bronchospasm, antinuclear antibodies, arthritis, myalgia, arthralgia, lupus-like syndrome, pulmonary complications	Not used
Hypotension, heart block, heart failure, bronchospasm, pain at infusion site	Not used
Heart block, heart failure, hypotension, asystole, dizziness, headache, fatigue, edema, nausea, constipation	Not used
Hypotension, heart block, asystole, heart failure	Not used
ORAL AMIODARONE: Pulmonary fibrosis, bradycardia, heart block, torsades de pointes (unusual), hyper- or hypothyroidism, GI upset, alcoholic-like hepatitis, peripheral neuropathy, ataxia, tremor, dizziness, photosensitivity, blue-gray skin, corneal microdeposits, optic neuritis IV AMIODARONE: Hypotension, bradycardia, phlebitis at site of administration	1 to 2 µg/ml (usefulness for monitoring toxicity unclear)

(continued)

Drug	Usual dosage* and interval	Effect on ECG
Sotalol (*Betapace*, and others)	80-160 mg twice daily (Higher doses can be used, but may be associated with increased adverse effects including torsades de pointes. Lower doses must be used in renal dysfunction)	Prolongs QT Sinus bradycardia
Dofetilide *(Tikosyn)*	125-500 μg bid (Lower doses must be used in renal dysfunction)	Prolongs QT

QUINIDINE, PROCAINAMIDE, DISOPYRAMIDE

Drug	Usual dosage* and interval	Effect on ECG
Quinidine (many manufacturers)	PO: 200-400 mg q4-6h (sulfate) 324-648 mg q8-12h (gluconate)	Prolongs QRS, QT and (±) PR
Procainamide (*Pronestyl, Procanbid*, and others)	PO: 50-100 mg/kg/day in divided doses, q3-4h or q6h (sustained-release) or q12h (extended-release) IV Loading: 20 mg/min (up to 17 mg/kg) IV Maintenance: 2-4 mg/min	Prolongs QRS, QT and (±) PR
Disopyramide (*Norpace*, and others)	PO: 100-200 mg q6-8h or 150-300 mg q12h (long-acting formulation)	Prolongs QRS, QT and (±) PR

FLECAINIDE, PROPAFENONE, MORICIZINE

Drug	Usual dosage* and interval	Effect on ECG
Flecainide‡ *(Tambocor)*	PO Initial dose: 50-100 mg q12h, increase q4 days if required, by 50 mg q12h PO Maintenance: ≤400 mg/day Cardioversion: 300 mg single dose PO***	Prolongs PR and QRS
Propafenone‡ *(Rythmol)*	PO Initial dose: 150 mg q8h, increase q3-4 days if required PO Maintenance: 150 to 300 mg q8h Cardioversion: 600 mg single dose PO***	Prolongs PR and QRS

   * Patients with decreased hepatic or renal function may require lower dosage.
  ** Not reliable due to saturable protein binding.
 *** Patients should also receive an AV nodal blocking agent such as verapamil, diltiazem or a beta-blocker.
   † Range of usually effective and tolerated concentrations
   ‡ Should not be used in patients with congestive heart failure or ischemic heart disease.

Adverse effects	Serum concentrations[†]
Heart block, hypotension, bronchospasm, bradycardia, torsades de pointes	0.5-1.0 µg/ml for beta-blockade, higher for QT effect (generally not clinically useful)
Torsades de pointes	Not used
Diarrhea and other GI symptoms, cinchonism, hepatic granulomas and necrosis, thrombocytopenia, rash, hypotension, heart block, ventricular tachyarrhythmias, torsades de pointes, fever, lupus-like syndrome	1.5 to 5 µg/ml
Lupus-like syndrome, confusion, disorientation, GI symptoms, rash, hypotension, ventricular arrhythmias, torsades de pointes, blood dyscrasias, fever, rare muscular weakness IV: hypotension, heart block	4 to 10 µg/ml (NAPA active metabolite: 7 to 15 µg/ml)
Anticholinergic effects (urinary retention, aggravation of glaucoma, constipation), hypotension, heart failure, ventricular tachyarrhythmias, torsades de pointes, heart block, nausea, vomiting, diarrhea, hypoglycemia, nervousness	2 to 5 µg/ml**
Bradycardia, heart block, new ventricular fibrillation, sustained ventricular tachycardia, heart failure, dizziness, blurred vision, nervousness, headache, GI upset, neutropenia	0.2 to 1 µg/ml
Bradycardia, heart block, new ventricular fibrillation, sustained ventricular tachycardia, heart failure, dizziness, lightheadedness, metallic taste, GI upset, bronchospasm, hepatic toxicity	Not established due to active metabolites

(continued)

Drug	Usual dosage* and interval	Effect on ECG
Moricizine (Ethmozine)	PO Initial dose: 200 mg q8h, increase by 150 mg/day q3-4 days if required PO Maintenance: 200-300 mg q8h	Prolongs PR and QRS

ADENOSINE

Drug	Usual dosage* and interval	Effect on ECG
Adenosine (Adenocard)	IV: 6 mg by rapid IV push followed by a saline flush; may use 12 mg for repeat rapid bolus injection	Prolongs PR Heart block (transient)

LIDOCAINE AND SIMILAR AGENTS

Drug	Usual dosage* and interval	Effect on ECG
Lidocaine (Xylocaine, and others)	IV Loading: 1 mg/kg given over 2 min, then 0.5 mg/kg over 2 min every 8-10 min x 3 or: 20 mg/min infused over 10 min IV Maintenance: 1-4 mg/min	No significant change
Mexiletine (Mexitil)	PO Initial dose: 150-200 mg q8h taken with food PO Maintenance: 150-300 mg q6-12h, maximum 1200 mg/day	No significant change
Tocainide (Tonocard)	PO Initial dose: 400 mg q8h with food PO Maintenance: 200-600 mg q8h, maximum 2400 mg/day	No significant change

OTHER AGENTS

Drug	Usual dosage* and interval	Effect on ECG
Bretylium	IV Loading: 5 mg/kg with additional doses of 10 mg/kg to maximum of 30 mg/kg (effect may be delayed) IV Maintenance: 5-10 mg/kg q6h or continuous infusion 1-2 mg/min	No change Sinus bradycardia
Digoxin (Lanoxin, and others)	IV or PO Loading: 1-1.5 mg over 24 hours in 3-4 divided doses Maintenance: 0.125-0.5 mg/day	Prolongs PR Depresses ST segment Flattens T wave
Ibutilide (Corvert)	IV: 1 mg over 10 minutes; may repeat once after a 10 minute wait	Prolongs QT
Magnesium	IV: 1-2 gm as $MgSO_4$	

* Patients with decreased hepatic or renal function may require lower dosage.

† Range of usually effective and tolerated concentrations

Adverse effects	Serum concentrations[†]
Bradycardia, heart failure, new ventricular fibrillation, sustained ventricular tachycardia, nausea, dizziness, headache	Not established due to active metabolites
Facial flushing, transient dyspnea, chest discomfort (non-coronary), hypotension; may cause broncho-constriction in patients with asthma	Not established
Drowsiness or agitation, slurred speech, tinnitus, disorientation, coma, seizures, paresthesias, cardiac depression, especially with excessive accumulation in heart failure or liver failure or infusions for more than 24 hours, bradycardia/asystole	1.5 to 5 µg/ml
GI upset, fatigue, nervousness, dizziness, tremor, sleep upset, seizures, visual disturbances, psychosis, fever, blood dyscrasias, hepatitis	0.5 to 2 µg/ml
GI upset, paresthesias, dizziness, tremor, confusion, nightmares, psychotic reactions, coma, seizures, rash, fever, arthralgia, agranulocytosis, aplastic anemia, thrombocytopenia, hepatic granulomas, interstitial pneumonitis	3 to 10 µg/ml
Orthostatic hypotension, nausea and vomiting, increased sensitivity to catecholamines, initial increase in arrhythmias	Not established
Bradycardia, AV block, arrhythmias, anorexia, nausea, vomiting, diarrhea, abdominal pain, headache, confusion, abnormal vision	0.8-2 ng/ml
Torsades de pointes	Not useful
Areflexia, respiratory depression, bradycardia, AV block, asystole with high doses	Not useful

FLECAINIDE, PROPAFENONE AND MORICIZINE — Flecainide *(Tambocor)*, and **propafenone** *(Rythmol)* markedly decrease the speed of cardiac conduction, but only modestly increase the ventricular refractory period. **Moricizine** *(Ethmozine)* also slows conduction and has little effect on repolarization. Although all three drugs are effective in suppressing ventricular arrhythmias, they also can aggravate existing arrhythmias or precipitate new ones, especially in patients with underlying heart disease and sustained ventricular tachycardia. Use of flecainide, encainide (no longer marketed) or moricizine in a clinical trial in post-myocardial infarction patients with asymptomatic ventricular arrhythmias was associated with an increase in mortality compared to placebo (AE Epstein et al, JAMA 1993; 270:2451). Whether propafenone, which unlike flecainide or moricizine also has beta-blocking activity in some patients, would have the same effect is unknown. Both propafenone and flecainide are effective in preventing episodes of paroxysmal supraventricular tachycardia and atrial fibrillation in patients with otherwise healthy hearts. Single large oral doses of propafenone or flecainide have been used to terminate atrial fibrillation (G Boriani et al, Ann Intern Med 1997; 126:621), but can rarely increase ventricular rate if an AV nodal blocking drug such as verapamil, diltiazem or a beta-blocker is not used concurrently.

ADENOSINE — Given intravenously, the nucleoside adenosine *(Adenocard)* is highly effective in terminating many supraventricular arrhythmias, although not multifocal atrial tachycardia or atrial fibrillation or flutter (LI Ganz and PL Friedman, N Engl J Med 1995; 332:162). Although it can cause heart block, hypotension, transient atrial fibrillation and chest discomfort, adenosine is probably safer than verapamil or diltiazem because it disappears from the circulation within seconds. Because of its safety, most cardiologists now prefer adenosine over a calcium-channel blocker for termination of sustained supraventricular tachycardia. As with calcium-channel blockers or digoxin, patients with Wolff-Parkinson-White syndrome who are in atrial fibrillation may develop serious ventricular arrhythmias when given standard doses of adenosine (DV Exner et al, Ann Intern Med 1995; 122:351).

LIDOCAINE AND SIMILAR AGENTS — Lidocaine *(Xylocaine*, and others), which is only given IV, is mainly metabolized by the liver.

Patients with heart failure or with decreased hepatic function and those more than 70 years old should receive lower maintenance doses. Clearance of the drug often decreases during therapy; monitoring plasma concentrations can decrease toxicity. Propranolol or cimetidine (*Tagamet*, and others) can decrease the clearance of lidocaine, and concurrent use of tocainide or mexiletine can cause additive CNS toxicity, including seizures. The practice of giving lidocaine prophylactically to patients with suspected acute myocardial infarction has largely been abandoned because clinical trials failed to show a reduction in mortality. Current CPR guidelines have replaced lidocaine with amiodarone as first-line therapy for ventricular arrhythmias causing cardiac arrest (Guidelines, Circulation 2000; 102 suppl I:I86).

Mexiletine *(Mexitil)* and **tocainide** *(Tonocard)* are orally effective congeners of lidocaine. Nausea and tremor are common with both drugs; nausea is less severe when the drugs are taken with food. Tocainide is rarely indicated because of adverse hematological effects, including a 0.2% incidence of agranulocytosis; it should be reserved for symptomatic patients who have not responded to other drugs, and blood counts should be monitored.

OTHER AGENTS — **Bretylium** given intravenously can stabilize cardiac rhythm in about 50% of patients with resistant ventricular fibrillation or recurrent ventricular tachycardia refractory to other treatment. **Digoxin** (*Lanoxin*, and others) can control ventricular response in atrial fibrillation or flutter and may terminate some paroxysmal (re-entrant) supraventricular arrhythmias, but other drugs may be more effective. Digoxin, like verapamil and diltiazem, is contraindicated for use in atrial fibrillation in patients with the Wolff-Parkinson-White syndrome. Intravenous **magnesium** appears to be effective in preventing recurrent drug-induced torsades de pointes and in some arrhythmias related to digitalis toxicity. **Ibutilide** *(Corvert)* is given intravenously for termination of atrial fibrillation or flutter (KT Murray, Circulation 1998; 97:493). It is effective in about 60% of patients with atrial flutter and 30% with atrial fibrillation. QT prolongation and torsades de pointes can occur; the incidence of torsades is about 1% to 3%, but higher in women.

NONPHARMACOLOGIC APPROACHES — **Radiofrequency (RF) catheter ablation** is a technique in which small areas of tissue responsible for the genesis or maintenance of some arrhythmias can be identified and destroyed (F Morady, N Engl J Med 1999; 340:534). **Implantable cardioverter/defibrillators (ICDs)** can be used in patients who have survived an episode of sustained ventricular tachycardia or fibrillation (Medical Letter 1994; 36:86). Three large randomized trials have compared ICD therapy to antiarrhythmic drugs (mainly amiodarone) in patients resuscitated from cardiac arrest or sustained ventricular tachycardia. One found better survival with an ICD (The Antiarrhythmics Versus Implantable Defibrillators (AVID) Investigators, N Engl J Med 1997; 337:1576), while the other two (K-H Kuck et al, Circulation 2000; 102:748; SJ Connolly et al, Circulation 2000; 101:1297) found a similar trend. In asymptomatic high-risk patients with arrhythmias inducible by programmed electrical stimulation of the heart, a large randomized study found lower mortality in patients with ICDs compared to those receiving antiarrhythmic drugs (AE Buxton et al, N Engl J Med 1999; 341:1882). In many of these trials, patients receiving ICDs had a higher rate of beta-blocker use, which may have contributed to the observed ICD effect. In high-risk asymptomatic patients undergoing coronary bypass, an ICD did not decrease mortality (JT Bigger, Jr et al, N Engl J Med 1997; 337:1569).

DRUGS FOR DEPRESSION AND ANXIETY

An ever-increasing number of drugs are available for treatment of depression, and most antidepressants are also effective for treatment of anxiety disorders. Adverse effects of these drugs are listed in the table beginning on page 81. Interactions with other drugs can be found in *The Medical Letter Handbook of Adverse Drug Interactions*, 2001. All antidepressants can cause mania, particularly in patients with bipolar disorder.

DOSAGE AND COST OF SOME DRUGS FOR DEPRESSION AND ANXIETY

Drug	Usual daily dosage	Cost[1]
SSRIs		
Citalopram – *Celexa* (Forest)	20 mg once/day	$ 61.80
Fluoxetine – *Prozac* (Lilly/Dista)	20 mg once/day	77.40
Prozac Weekly	90 mg once/week	73.80
Paroxetine – *Paxil* (GlaxoSmithKline)	20 mg once/day	71.40
Sertraline – *Zoloft* (Pfizer)	100 mg once/day	69.60
Tricyclic Antidepressants		
Amitriptyline – average generic price	150 mg once/day	13.50
Elavil (AstraZeneca)		61.80
Desipramine – average generic price	150 mg once/day	25.20
Norpramin (Aventis)		97.50
Imipramine – generic	150 mg once/day	32.40
Tofranil (Novartis)		91.80
Tofranil PM		80.40
Nortriptyline – generic	75 mg once/day	27.30
Pamelor (Novartis)		107.40
MAOIs		
Phenelzine – *Nardil* (Parke-Davis)	30 mg b.i.d.	61.20
Tranylcypromine – *Parnate* (GlaxoSmithKline)	20 mg b.i.d.	70.80
Other Antidepressants		
Bupropion – average generic price	100 mg t.i.d.	79.20
Wellbutrin (GlaxoSmithKline)		95.40
Wellbutrin SR	150 mg b.i.d.	91.80
Mirtazapine – *Remeron* (Organon)	30 mg once/day	76.50
Remeron Sol Tab		70.50

(continued)

1. Average cost to the patient for a 30-day supply, based on data from retail pharmacies nationwide, provided by Scott-Levin's *Source*™ *Prescription Audit (SPA)*, May 2000 to April 2001.

Drug	Usual daily dosage	Cost[1]
Other Antidepressants (continued)		
Nefazodone – *Serzone* (Bristol-Myers Squibb)	200 mg b.i.d.	$73.80
Trazodone – average generic price	300 mg in divided doses	35.10
Desyrel (Apothecon)		309.60
Desyrel Dividose		153.30
Venlafaxine – *Effexor* (Wyeth-Ayerst)	75 mg b.i.d.	80.40
Effexor XR	150 mg once/day	74.10
Benzodiazepines for Anxiety		
Alprazolam – averge generic price	0.5 mg q.i.d.[2]	37.20
Xanax (Pharmacia)		134.40
Clonazepam – average generic price	0.5 mg b.i.d.[2]	30.00
Klonopin (Roche)		49.20
Diazepam – average generic price	10 mg b.i.d.	13.20
Valium (Roche)		85.20
Lorazepam – average generic price	1 mg t.i.d.	57.60
Ativan (Wyeth-Ayerst)		96.30
Oxazepam – average generic price	15 mg t.i.d.	54.90
Serax (Faulding)		100.80
Other Anti-Anxiety Drugs		
Buspirone – average generic price	15 mg b.i.d.	112.20
BuSpar Dividose (Bristol-Myers Squibb)		123.00

2. Patients with panic disorder often require higher dosage.

DRUGS FOR DEPRESSION — Most antidepressants are effective in about 50% to 60% of patients with major depression, but 80% or more of patients will respond to at least one antidepressant drug (MA Whooley and GE Simon, N Engl J Med 2000; 343:1942). Maintenance therapy is recommended for patients with recurrent depression because of their high risk of recurrence. Antidepressant drugs are also helpful for some patients with dysthymia, a chronic low-level form of depression (JW Williams et al, Ann Intern Med 2000; 132:743). Treatment of depression complicated by psychosis requires an antidepressant and an antipsychotic drug. Electroconvulsive therapy (ECT) remains an effective treatment that may be useful in severe depression, delusional depression, in elderly patients who may not be able to tolerate drugs, and in patients who do not respond to drugs.

Choice of Drugs – Antidepressants often take about two weeks to produce improvement, may take as long as six weeks to achieve substantial benefit, and may take longer for maximum benefit (AJ Gelenberg and CL Chesen, J Clin Psychiatry 2000; 61:712). Because of their more tolerable adverse effects and relative safety in overdose, newer antidepressants such as the selective serotonin reuptake inhibitors (SSRIs) have largely replaced the older tricyclics and monoamine oxidase inhibitors (MAOIs) as first-line drugs. Nevertheless, tricyclics and MAOIs remain valuable alternatives for patients with moderate to severe depression.

Venlafaxine, bupropion, nefazodone and mirtazapine are sometimes selected as first-line drugs for their particular clinical profiles. The sleep-enhancing effects of nefazodone and sedative effects of mirtazapine can be useful when insomnia or agitation are prominent. The appetite-increasing effects of mirtazapine may be advantageous particularly in depressed elderly patients with marked anorexia. The absence of sexual dysfunction, weight gain or sedation with bupropion may be beneficial for patients who cannot tolerate other drugs. Trazodone has been considered a less effective antidepressant but is frequently used adjunctively for SSRI-associated sleep disturbances. Severe premenstrual dysphoric symptoms have been treated successfully with the SSRIs; fluoxetine *(Sarafem)* is FDA-approved for this indication (Medical Letter 2001; 43:5). St. John's wort is an over-the-counter herbal extract widely used for treatment of depression; one multicenter controlled trial found no statisticaaly significant advantage over placebo (RC Shelton et al, JAMA 2000; 285:1978).

When patients show only a partial response to an antidepressant, some experts add a second drug, such as lithium, for "augmentation" or combine two antidepressants of different classes, such as an SSRI and bupropion (JC Nelson, J Clin Psychiatry 2000; 61 suppl 2:13).

Adverse Effects – The most common adverse effects associated with the **SSRIs** are nausea, diarrhea, headache, nervousness, insomnia, fatigue and sexual dysfunction. Jitteriness and insomnia early in treatment can be minimized by beginning with low doses or giving the drug in the morning. The SSRIs are much less likely to produce orthostatic hypotension and anticholinergic effects than are the tricyclics. Paroxetine can, however, have mild anticholinergic effects. The SSRIs appear to be safer than tricyclics in patients with heart disease (SP Roose et al, JAMA 1998; 279:287), and they are much safer in overdose. Weight gain can occur with prolonged use. Sexual dysfunction (including decreased libido, impaired arousal and anorgasmia) is a common adverse effect and may affect a majority of patients treated with SSRIs. Withdrawal effects when SSRIs are discontinued include dizziness, nausea, paresthesias, tremor, anxiety and dysphoria; they can be minimized by gradual tapering and are least likely to occur with fluoxetine, which has the longest half-life (PM Haddad, Drug Saf 2001; 24:183). SSRIs interact with many other drugs (*The Medical Letter Handbook of Adverse Drug Interactions*, 2001, page 413); sertraline and citalopram may be least likely to interact.

Venlafaxine is similar to the SSRIs in its adverse effects but is more likely to cause nausea and at higher doses can cause a dose-dependent increase in diastolic blood pressure. A withdrawal syndrome can occur with rapid dose reductions, or even after missing a single day's dose, and may be more severe than with SSRIs. The most common adverse effects of **nefazodone** are somnolence, dry mouth, nausea and dizziness; jitteriness, sexual dysfunction and sleep disturbance generally do not occur. Nefazodone is a potent inhibitor of CYP3A4 and can potentiate the effects of alprazolam (*Xanax*, and others), triazolam (*Halcion*, and others) or midazolam (*Versed*, and others), and may lead to QT prolongation when co-administered with pimozide *(Orap)*. The most common adverse effects of **trazodone** are sedation, orthostatic hypotension and nausea; rarely it can cause priapism, potentially leading to permanent loss of erectile function. Sedation, increased appetite, weight gain, dizziness, dry mouth and constipation can occur with **mirtazapine**. **Bupropion** can cause agitation, anxiety, insomnia, headache, nausea and, rarely, dose-related seizures; it is contraindicated in patients thought to have an increased risk of seizures. Bupropion is unlikely to cause weight gain, sexual dysfunction, anticholinergic effects, hypotension or cardiac effects.

Tricyclic antidepressants commonly cause anticholinergic effects (urinary retention, constipation, dry mouth, and blurred vision), orthostatic hypotension, weight gain, sedation and sexual dysfunction. Elderly patients are more sensitive to the anticholinergic effects of tricyclics and may develop confusion or delirium. Nortriptyline and desipramine cause fewer anticholinergic effects and less sedation than amitriptyline or imipramine. Orthostatic hypotension in the elderly may lead to falls; it is least likely to occur with nortriptyline. Tricyclics also have ion-channel-blocking effects on the heart; another class of antidepressant is preferred for patients with cardiac conduction abnormalities or ischemic heart disease. Accidental or intentional overdosage with as little as a one-week supply of a tricyclic can cause hypotension, seizures, cardiac arrhythmias, coma and death. Withdrawal symptoms (sleep disturbance, nightmares, malaise, gastrointestinal upset, and irritability) have been reported with abrupt discontinuation of a tricyclic after long-term use.

Adverse effects commonly associated with the **MAO inhibitors** (MAOIs) include sleep disturbance, orthostatic hypotension, sexual dysfunction, and weight gain as well as dangerous and even fatal interactions with certain other drugs and foods. Concurrent use of sympathomimetic agents, including levodopa and over-the-counter drugs marketed as decongestants, stimulants or weight loss aids can precipitate a hypertensive crisis. Foods high in tyramine can also precipitate a hypertensive crisis in patients taking an MAOI (*The Medical Letter Handbook of Adverse Drug Interactions* 2001, page 445). Some clinicians prescribe nifedipine (*Adalat*, and others) 10 to 20 mg for emergency self-administration if that should happen. Concomitant use of serotonergic agents such as an SSRI, clomipramine (*Anafranil*, and others), analgesics such as tramadol (*Ultram*), or the cough-suppressant dextromethophan can produce a "serotonin syndrome" characterized by hyperpyrexia, confusion, agitation, neuromuscular irritability, hypotension, coma and death. Triptans, except naratriptan (*Amerge*), are contraindicated while taking an MAO inhibitor and for two weeks after stopping one. Concomitant use of meperidine (*Demerol*, and others) with an MAO inhibitor can cause severe encephalopathy and death. A drug-free interval of two weeks is recommended when switching from an MAOI to another MAOI or another antidepressant. A drug-free interval of one or two weeks is recommended when switching from an SSRI to an MAOI, except that a patient who has been taking fluoxetine should wait at least five weeks before beginning an MAOI.

St. John's wort is generally well tolerated but may lower plasma concentrations of some other drugs including oral contraceptives, cyclosporine (*Sandimmune*, and others), warfarin (*Coumadin*, and others), indinavir *(Crixivan)* and theophylline, or increase toxicity when used concomitantly with other antidepressants (Medical Letter 2000; 42:56).

Use in Pregnancy – Maternal depression itself may be associated with intrauterine growth problems or low birth weight, so the risks of exposure to antidepressants during pregnancy must be weighed against the risks of untreated depression. MAO inhibitors have been associated with a few cases of teratogenicity. Studies of tricyclics and SSRIs have not found evidence of teratogenicity or intrauterine death, but extensive data on other classes of antidepressants are lacking. Fluoxetine, the most extensively studied SSRI in pregnancy, does not appear to be associated with major malformations, growth impairment or behavioral problems. In one prospective non-randomized study, third trimester exposure to fluoxetine was associated with lower birth weight and perinatal complications, but a causal relationship could not be established (CD Chambers et al, N Engl J Med 1996; 335:1010). SSRIs and tricyclics have been associated with a neonatal withdrawal syndrome (KL Wisner et al, JAMA 2000; 282:1264).

DRUGS FOR ANXIETY — For most patients with an anxiety disorder, antidepressants are the drugs of first choice because depression and anxiety frequently co-exist. It is not clear, however, whether bupropion has antianxiety properties. As in the treatment of depression, these drugs may take several weeks to act.

All benzodiazepines appear to be equally effective for most forms of anxiety, but pharmacokinetic differences may be important. The anticonvulsant gabapentin *(Neurontin)* has also been used for anxiety disorders as a nonabusable alternative to benzodiazepines, even though evidence for its efficacy is limited.

Generalized anxiety disorder can be treated with an antidepressant, a benzodiazepine or buspirone. Only venlafaxine and paroxetine have been approved by the FDA for treatment of generalized anxiety disorder, but other SSRIs, tricyclics and nefazodone have also been effective. Fluvoxamine *(Luvox)*, an SSRI FDA-approved only for treatment of obsessive-compulsive disorder, was effective in a placebo-controlled eight-week trial for treatment of generalized anxiety disorder, separation anxiety disorder and social phobia in children and adolescents (Research Unit on Pediatric Psychopharmacology Anxiety Study Group, N Engl J Med 2001; 344:1279). Buspirone is nonsedating and not addicting, but it may take up to four weeks to act, and some Medical Letter consultants have found it less effective than the benzodiazepines.

Panic disorder can be effectively treated with antidepressants. Because of their safety and tolerability, the SSRIs are considered the drugs of first choice for this disorder, but tricyclics and MAOIs are also effective. Many clinicians prescribing an SSRI or tricyclic antidepressant for this indication begin with low doses to avoid an initial increase in anxiety. A benzodiazepine such as clonazepam, which is potent and long-acting, provides rapid relief of symptoms and can be used alone to treat panic disorder in patients who do not have a history of substance abuse and are not depressed. Alprazolam, although widely used, may cause rebound anxiety between doses and can be difficult to discontinue. Other drugs that have been effective for panic disorder in some patients include venlafaxine, nefazodone and gabapentin.

Social phobia can be successfully treated with an SSRI or MAOI. Propranolol *(Inderal*, and others) and other beta-blockers have been used PRN to prevent symptoms of **performance anxiety** ("stage fright"). Drug treatment is usually not recommended for treatment of **specific phobias** such as fear of heights, flying, animals or closed spaces; behavior therapy is the treatment of choice for these disorders.

Serotonergic antidepressants such as clomipramine *(Anafranil*, and others), and the SSRIs fluvoxamine, fluoxetine, paroxetine, sertraline and citalopram are the drugs of choice for **obsessive-**

compulsive disorder, but higher doses than those used to treat depression may be required. Partial relief of obsessive-compulsive symptoms may develop gradually over several weeks or months; treatment should be continued for at least 10 weeks before these drugs are considered ineffective. Patients who do not respond to one of these drugs may respond to another.

Posttraumatic stress disorder (PTSD) is characterized by intrusive memories and nightmares, emotional numbing, avoidance behavior and hyperarousal symptoms following traumatic events. The SSRIs are considered first-line drugs for this disorder; sertraline has been shown to be effective (K Brady et al, JAMA 2000; 283:1837) and is approved by the FDA for treatment of PTSD. Other drugs that have been helpful for some symptoms of PTSD include nefazodone, MAOIs and valproate. Drug treatment without psychotherapy is not recommended.

Adverse Effects – Sedation is the most common adverse effect of the **benzodiazepines** and may increase mental confusion and the risk of falls in the elderly. Ataxia, anterograde amnesia or behavioral disinhibition may occur in some patients. Respiratory depression can occur in patients with underlying pulmonary disease. Oral overdoses of benzodiazepines are rarely lethal unless combined with other central nervous system depressants such as alcohol, barbiturates or opioids. Flumazenil *(Romazicon)* is an effective antidote for benzodiazepine oversedation. With **buspirone**, headache, dizziness, and nausea are the most common adverse effects. **Gabapentin** can produce somnolence, fatigue, dizziness, ataxia, nystagmus and tremor.

Withdrawal – Physical dependence may develop with chronic use of benzodiazepines. Rebound anxiety and withdrawal symptoms (insomnia, nausea, vomiting, twitching, irritability, paresthesias, tinnitus, delirium and, occasionally, seizures) may occur with abrupt or rapid discontinuation. Withdrawal symptoms are most likely after discontinuation of shorter-acting benzodiazepines such as alprazolam and lorazepam. Tapering of dosage, sometimes over weeks or months, is recommended. Buspirone has not been associated with physical dependence or withdrawal and will not block symptoms of benzodiazepine withdrawal.

Use in Pregnancy – A meta-analysis of benzodiazepine use during pregnancy found little evidence of risk but could not rule out an association with cleft lip or palate (LR Dolovich et al, BMJ 1998; 317:839). No adequate studies of buspirone or gabapentin in pregnancy are available.

ADVERSE EFFECTS OF SOME DRUGS FOR DEPRESSION AND ANXIETY

ALPRAZOLAM (*Xanax*, and others), see Benzodiazepines

AMITRIPTYLINE (*Elavil*, and others), see Tricyclic antidepressants

AMOXAPINE (*Asendin*, and others), see Tricyclic antidepressants

BENZODIAZEPINES (alprazolam, chlordiazepoxide, clonazepam, clorazepate, diazepam, halazepam, lorazepam, oxazepam)
Frequent: Drowsiness; ataxia
Occasional: Confusion; amnesia; disinhibition; paradoxical excitement; depression; dizziness; withdrawal symptoms, including delirium and convulsions, on abrupt discontinuance (withdrawal may be especially difficult with alprazolam); rebound insomnia or excitement
Rare: Hypotension; blood dyscrasias; jaundice; allergic reactions; paradoxical rage reactions; respiratory depression in patients with pulmonary disease

BUPROPION (*Wellbutrin*)
Frequent: Anxiety; agitation; insomnia; tremor; anorexia; constipation; nausea; dry mouth; headache
Occasional: Sweating; tinnitus; rash
Rare: Seizures (dose-related); mania; psychosis; serum sickness-like reaction

BUSPIRONE (*BuSpar*)
Frequent: Dizziness; headache
Occasional: Nausea; paresthesias; diarrhea
Rare: Psychosis; mania

CHLORDIAZEPOXIDE (*Librium*, and others), see Benzodiazepines

CITALOPRAM (*Celexa*), see Selective Serotonin Reuptake Inhibitors

CLOMIPRAMINE (*Anafranil*, and others), see Tricyclic antidepressants

CLONAZEPAM (*Klonopin*, and others), see Benzodiazepines

CLORAZEPATE (*Tranxene*, and others), see Benzodiazepines

DESIPRAMINE (*Norpramin*, and others), see Tricyclic antidepressants

DIAZEPAM (*Valium*, and others), see Benzodiazepines

DOXEPIN (*Adapin*, and others), see Tricyclic antidepressants

FLUOXETINE (*Prozac*), see Selective Serotonin Reuptake Inhibitors

FLUVOXAMINE (*Luvox*), see Selective Serotonin Reuptake Inhibitors

GABAPENTIN (*Neurontin*)
  Frequent: Somnolence; fatigue; dizziness; ataxia; nystagmus; tremor
  Occasional: Weight gain; arthralgia; edema; dyspepsia; depression; irritability; diplopia; blurred vision
  Rare: choreoathetosis; oculogyric crisis

IMIPRAMINE (*Tofranil*, and others), see Tricyclic antidepressants

LORAZEPAM (*Ativan*, and others), see Benzodiazepines

MAO INHIBITORS (isocarboxazid, phenelzine, tranylcypromine)
  Frequent: Postural hypotension with phenelzine; restlessness; insomnia; daytime sleepiness
  Occasional: Mania; urinary retention; tremors; sexual disturbances; paresthesias; dry mouth; nausea; constipation; anorexia; weight gain; edema; withdrawal symptoms
  Rare: Rash; hepatitis; tinnitus; muscle spasm; lupus-like reaction; leukopenia; hyperthermia; hypertension (Note: Interactions with drugs or tyramine-containing foods may be severe)

MIRTAZAPINE (*Remeron*)
  Frequent: Somnolence; weight gain; increased appetite; dizziness; dry mouth; constipation
  Occasional: Asthenia; increased aminotransferase activity; increased cholesterol/triglycerides
  Rare: Mania; agranulocytosis; sexual dysfunction

NEFAZODONE (*Serzone*)
  Frequent: Somnolence; headache; dizziness; dry mouth; nausea
  Occasional: Confusion; constipation; dyspepsia; postural hypotension; abnormal vision
  Rare: Sexual dysfunction; mania; akathisia; hepatic failure

NORTRIPTYLINE (*Aventyl*, and others), see Tricyclic antidepressants

OXAZEPAM (*Serax*, and others), see Benzodiazepines

PAROXETINE (*Paxil*), see Selective Serotonin Reuptake Inhibitors

PHENELZINE (*Nardil*), see MAO inhibitors

PROTRIPTYLINE (*Vivactil*), see Tricyclic antidepressants

SELECTIVE SEROTONIN REUPTAKE INHIBITORS (citalopram, fluoxetine, fluvoxamine, paroxetine, sertraline)
  Frequent: Nausea; headache; diarrhea; agitation; insomnia; drowsiness; dizziness; tremor; fatigue; increased sweating; sexual dysfunction; withdrawal reactions with sudden discontinuation (dizziness, paresthesias, headache, nausea, insomnia, anxiety)

Occasional: Dry mouth; anxiety; mania; indifference and apathy; paresthesias; anorexia; palpitations; increased urinary frequency; hot flushes; weight gain with prolonged use; constipation; blurred vision; mammoplasia; abulia; dyspepsia; alopecia; postural hypotension with paroxetine

Rare: Rhinitis; cognitive dysfunction; rash; yawning; myalgia; hypoesthesia; taste disturbances; tinnitus; thirst; extrapyramidal reactions; galactorrhea; platelet dysfunction and bleeding; inappropriate ADH secretion; bradycardia with syncope; seizures; serum sickness; pulmonary phospholipidosis; leukocytosis; hepatic toxicity; aplastic anemia with fluoxetine; penile anesthesia; bruxism

SERTRALINE (*Zoloft*), see Selective Serotonin Reuptake Inhibitors

TRANYLCYPROMINE (*Parnate*), see MAO inhibitors

TRAZODONE (*Desyrel*, and others)
Frequent: Drowsiness; headache; gastrointestinal upset
Occasional: Ventricular arrhythmias; peripheral edema; postural hypotension
Rare: Priapism; increased libido

TRICYCLIC ANTIDEPRESSANTS (amitriptyline, amoxapine, clomipramine, desipramine, doxepin, imipramine, nortriptyline, protriptyline, trimipramine)
Frequent: Anticholinergic effects;* orthostatic hypotension (less with nortriptyline); drowsiness; weight gain; tachycardia

Occasional: Mania; psychosis; tremor; first-degree heart block; other ECG abnormalities; rash; sweating; confusion; insomnia; anorgasmia and other sexual disturbances, especially with clomipramine; increase in dental caries; gingivitis; withdrawal symptoms

Rare: Hepatic toxicity; tinnitus; bone marrow depression, including agranulocytosis; peripheral neuropathy; severe cardiovascular effects in patients with cardiac disease; photosensitivity; dysarthria; stuttering; nausea, tremor, and seizures may be more common with clomipramine; extrapyramidal symptoms, tardive dyskinesia and neuroleptic malignant syndrome with amoxapine; renal failure with overdosage of amoxapine

TRIMIPRAMINE (*Surmontil*, and others), see Tricyclic antidepressants

VENLAFAXINE (*Effexor*)
Frequent: Nausea; somnolence; dizziness; headache; sweating; anorexia; insomnia; nervousness; anxiety; sexual dysfunction; withdrawal reactions with sudden discontinuation (dizziness, paresthesias, headache, nausea, insomnia, anxiety)
Occasional: Weight loss; dry mouth; constipation; dose-dependent increase in blood pressure
Rare: Increased QT interval; hypotension; seizures; increased ocular pressure; inappropriate ADH secretion

---

* Dry mouth, mydriasis, cycloplegia, urinary retention, decreased GI motility, tachycardia, memory impairment and, in high doses, delirium

DRUGS FOR EPILEPSY

Treatment of epilepsy should begin with a single drug, increasing the dosage gradually until seizures are controlled or adverse effects become unacceptable. If seizures continue and further dosage increases appear inadvisable because of adverse effects, most Medical Letter consultants generally prescribe at least one and sometimes a second alternative drug before considering use of two drugs at the same time. In some cases, add-on therapy may also be safe and effective (TR Browne and GL Holmes, N Engl J Med 2001; 344:1145; P Kwan and MJ Brodie, Seizure 2000; 9:464). Monitoring serum concentrations of the drugs is helpful (MJ Eadie, Br J Clin Pharmacol 1998; 46:185). Most antiepileptic drugs initially approved by the FDA only for adjunctive therapy are also effective as monotherapy. Many of the drugs used to treat epilepsy interact with each other and with other drugs; for details, see *The Medical Letter Handbook of Adverse Drug Interactions*, 2001. The treatment of status epilepticus is not included here.

CARBAMAZEPINE — Carbamazepine (*Tegretol*, and others) is available only for oral use. It is particularly effective for treatment of partial and secondarily generalized tonic-clonic seizures, but it may make absence or myoclonic seizures worse (P Genton et al, Neurology 2000; 55:1106). Carbamazepine induces its own metabolism; serum concentrations often fall after a few weeks of treatment. Therapeutic failure associated with poor bioavailability has been reported with both generic carbamazepine and with *Tegretol*, particularly when tablets are stored in humid conditions, which cause concretion of the tablets. Two extended-release formulations, *Carbatrol* and *Tegretol XR*, are now available.

Adverse Effects – Carbamazepine can cause dose-related rash, drowsiness, blurred vision, transient diplopia, headache, dizziness, ataxia, nausea and vomiting, and can interfere with cognitive function in learning situations. Mild leukopenia or hyponatremia are fairly common. With high doses of the drug, hypofibrinogenemia and thrombocytopenia can occur, but are usually reversible if the drug is discontinued. Agranulocytosis, aplastic anemia, cardiac toxicity, aseptic meningitis, intractable diarrhea, hepatitis and hypersensitivity reactions (including Stevens-Johnson syndrome), which can be fatal, are rare. Circulating concentrations of thyroid hormones may be depressed, while TSH remains normal. Abnormal color perception can occur (I Nousianen et al, Ophthalmology 2000; 107:884).

PHENYTOIN (diphenylhydantoin) — Phenytoin (*Dilantin*, and others) is as effective as carbamazepine for treatment of partial and secondarily generalized tonic-clonic seizures. Different formulations of phenytoin may not be bioequivalent. Fosphenytoin (*Cerebyx*) is a water soluble prodrug of phenytoin available for IV and IM use that does not cause soft tissue injury as older IV formulations do.

Adverse Effects – Nystagmus may occur with therapeutic serum concentrations of phenytoin and is nearly always present at higher concentrations. At total serum concentrations higher than 20 µg/ml, drowsiness, ataxia and diplopia may occur. Cerebellar atrophy has been reported even after acute intoxication (T Kuruvilla and NE Bharucha, Epilepsia 1997; 38:500; Z Alioglu et al, J Neuroradiol 2000; 27:52). Gingival hyperplasia, coarsening of facial features and hirsutism can be troublesome. A morbilliform or scarlatiniform rash may occur, usually in the first four weeks of treatment, sometimes with hepatitis, fever and lymphadenopathy; rarely it progresses to exfoliative dermatitis or Stevens-Johnson syndrome. Patients who develop rash with phenytoin are often susceptible to similar hypersensitivity reactions to carbamazepine and phenobarbital (AR Morkunas and MB Miller, Crit Care Clin 1997; 13:727). Phenytoin may interfere with cognitive function in learning situations. Less common adverse effects include megaloblastic anemia, a lupus-like syndrome, hepatic granulomas, hepatitis leading rarely to fatal hepatic necrosis, peripheral neuropathy, nephritis, and rickets and osteomalacia due to increased vitamin D metabolism. Serum folic acid, thyroxine and vitamin K concentrations may decrease with long-term therapy.

VALPROATE — Valproate, which is marketed as valproic acid (*Depakene*, and others) or divalproex sodium *(Depakote)*, is approved by the US Food and Drug Administration (FDA) for treatment of complex partial seizures, absence seizures and multiple seizure types that include absence seizures. The drug is also available for IV use *(Depacon)*. Because it is effective and usually well tolerated, valproate is also widely used for myoclonic, atonic and primary generalized tonic-clonic seizures. It is highly effective in treating photosensitive epilepsy and juvenile myoclonic epilepsy (GF Harding et al, Epilepsia 1997; 38:663; ST Wallace, Epilepsy Res 1998; 29:147). In one controlled trial, valproate was less effective than carbamazepine in controlling complex partial seizures, but equally effective for controlling secondarily generalized seizures (RH Mattson et al, N Engl J Med 1992; 327:765). A new extended-release formulation is available *(Depakote ER)* but is FDA-approved only for prophylactic treatment of migraine and is not bio-equivalent to delayed-release tablets.

Adverse Effects – Drowsiness due to valproate is usually mild and transient, and adverse cognitive effects are generally minimal. Nausea and vomiting can be minimized by using the enteric-coated formulation (*Depakote*), by taking the drug with food and by slow titration to an optimal dose. Weight gain is common in patients taking valproate, and has been associated with polycystic ovaries, hyperinsulinemia, lipid abnormalities, hirsutism and menstrual disturbances in women, and with increased serum androgen concentrations in men (V Biton et al, Neurology 2001; 56:172; JI Isojärvi et al, Ann Neurol 1998; 43:446; J Rättayä et al, Neurology 2001; 56:31). Dose-related tremor, transient hair loss and thrombocytopenia can also occur.

Serious adverse effects of the drug are uncommon, but fatal liver failure has occurred, particularly in children less than two years old taking valproate in combination with other anticonvulsants and in patients with developmental delay and metabolic disorders; liver failure has also been reported in older children and adults taking valproate alone. Even in the absence of hepatic dysfunction, valproate can interfere with conversion of ammonia to urea and infrequently causes lethargy associated with increased blood ammonia concentrations. Life-threatening pancreatitis, interstitial nephritis, reversible parkinsonism and edema requiring diuretics for control have occurred rarely.

PHENOBARBITAL AND PRIMIDONE— Phenobarbital and primidone (*Mysoline*, and others) are alternative drugs for treatment of generalized tonic-clonic seizures and partial seizures. The anticonvulsant effect of primidone is due both to the drug itself and its metabolites, which include phenobarbital; when monitoring is necessary, both primidone and phenobarbital concentrations should be measured. The half-life of phenobarbital is about 100 hours, and steady-state serum concentrations may not be reached for several weeks. Rapid absorption has made phenobarbital a common choice for treatment of seizures in infants, but adverse effects on cognitive function and school performance have led to decreased use in older children and adults. Cognitive effects are more severe with phenobarbital and primidone than with other antiepileptic drugs. The principal adverse effects of both drugs are sedation and behavior disturbances including hyperactivity, loss of concentration and depression. Hypersensitivity reactions similar to those produced by phenytoin and carbamazepine are rare but can be fatal.

ETHOSUXIMIDE — Ethosuximide (*Zarontin*) is recommended for treatment of uncomplicated absence seizures and is usually well tolerated. Adverse effects may include nausea, vomiting, lethargy, hiccups, headache and mood changes. Blood dyscrasias, erythema multiforme, Stevens-Johnson syndrome and a lupus-like syndrome have been reported. Psychotic behavior can occur. The elimination half-life is about 60 hours in adults, but only about 30 hours in children.

FELBAMATE — Felbamate (*Felbatol*) was approved by the FDA for use alone or with other drugs in adults with partial and secondarily generalized seizures and as adjunctive therapy in children with the multiple types of seizures associated with the Lennox-Gastaut syndrome. Aplastic anemia occurs with an incidence between 1:4000 and 1:5000, and is more common in patients with previous blood dyscrasias or autoimmune disease (JM Pellock,

Epilepsia 1999; 40 suppl 5:S57). This, in addition to reports of acute hepatic failure, has generally limited use of the drug to patients with severe refractory epilepsy.

GABAPENTIN — Gabapentin *(Neurontin)* is used for adjunctive therapy in adults and children with partial and secondarily generalized seizures, and is also effective as monotherapy (DW Chadwick et al, Neurology 1998; 51:1282; R Appleton et al, Epilepsia 1999; 40:1147). Like carbamazepine, gabapentin can exacerbate myoclonic seizures (J Asconape et al, Epilepsia 2000; 41:479). Gabapentin is not metabolized and is almost completely excreted by the kidneys. Dosage adjustment is required in patients with impaired renal function. Unlike other antiepileptic drugs, it does not induce or inhibit hepatic microsomal enzymes and does not affect the metabolism of other antiepileptic drugs taken concurrently. Gabapentin also is generally well tolerated. Adverse effects, which include somnolence, dizziness, ataxia, fatigue and nystagmus, are usually mild and often transient. Gabapentin can cause irritability, weight gain and behavioral changes in children, and has been associated with movement disorders (DO Lee et al, Epilepsia 1996; 37:87; AL Reeves et al, Epilepsia 1996; 37:988).

LAMOTRIGINE — Lamotrigine *(Lamictal)* is approved in the USA for adjunctive therapy or conversion to monotherapy in adults with partial seizures and as an adjunct in children and adults with Lennox-Gastaut syndrome (J Motte et al, N Engl J Med 1997; 337:1807; F Gilliam et al, Neurology 1998; 51:1018). It is also effective in other types of generalized seizures in both adults and children, although it can make myoclonus worse, particularly severe myoclonic epilepsy in infancy (A Biraben et al, Neurology 2000; 55:1758). In patients with newly diagnosed partial or generalized seizures, lamotrigine alone was as effective as carbamazepine or phenytoin, and better tolerated (MJ Brodie et al, Lancet 1995; 345:476; TJ Steiner et al, Epilepsia 1999; 40:601). When added to valproate therapy, the recommended dose is lower because valproate decreases clearance of lamotrigine. The most common adverse effects of lamotrigine include dizziness, ataxia, somnolence, headache, diplopia, nausea, vomiting and rash. Acute hepatitis has been reported (G Sauvé et al, Dig Dis Sci 2000;

45:1874). Severe, life-threatening rashes including Stevens-Johnson syndrome have occurred in about 0.3% of adults and about 1% of children in clinical trials (JA Messenheimer et al, Drug Saf 2000; 22:303). The risk may be increased by rapid increases in dosage or co-administration of valproate. The manufacturer recommends discontinuing the drug at the first sign of rash.

CLONAZEPAM — Clonazepam (*Klonopin,* and others) is a benzodiazepine used to treat myoclonic, atonic, and absence seizures resistant to treatment with other anticonvulsants. It is generally less effective for absence seizures than ethosuximide or valproate, and development of tolerance to its effects is common. Adverse effects of clonazepam include drowsiness, ataxia and behavior disorders. Withdrawal symptoms can occur after abrupt discontinuation.

TOPIRAMATE — Topiramate *(Topamax)* is approved as adjunctive therapy for partial and primary generalized tonic-clonic seizures in adults and children more than two years old. It is also effective in other types of seizures and in monotherapy (V Biton, Epilepsia 1997; 38 suppl 1:S42; RC Sachdeo, Clin Pharmacokinet 1998; 34:335). Topiramate has been effective in decreasing tonic and atonic seizures in children with Lennox-Gastaut syndrome (TA Glauser, Can J Neurol Sci 1998; 25:S8; RC Sachdeo et al, Neurology 1999; 52:1882). The drug is partly metabolized in the liver but is mostly excreted unchanged in the urine, so dosage reduction is required in patients with renal impairment. It usually does not significantly affect serum concentrations of other anticonvulsants taken concurrently, but in patients with high serum phenytoin concentrations may increase phenytoin levels by up to 25%. The most frequent adverse effects are drowsiness, dizziness, headache and ataxia. Nervousness, confusion, paresthesias and diplopia can occur. Psychomotor slowing, word-finding difficulty, impaired concentration, and interference with memory are common and may require stopping the drug. Low dosing and slow titration may minimize these effects (AP Aldenkamp et al, Epilepsia 2000; 41:1167). Weight loss is also common. Liver failure has been reported (K Bjøro et al, Lancet 1998; 352:1119; RJ Doan and M Clendennings, Can J Psychiatry 2000; 45:937). Renal stones have occurred, probably due to weak inhibition of carbonic anhydrase.

TIAGABINE — Tiagabine *(Gabitril)* is FDA-approved for use as adjunctive therapy in patients at least 12 years old with partial seizures, and is generally used only in these types of seizures (Medical Letter 1998; 40:45). Tiagabine inhibits γ-aminobutyric acid (GABA) uptake by neurons and glial cells; the resulting prolongation of action of this major inhibitory neurotransmitter is probably the mechanism of seizure control. Tiagabine is available for oral use only. It does not induce hepatic enzymes and therefore does not affect the concentrations of coadministered drugs such as carbamazepine or warfarin (*Coumadin*, and others). Tiagabine should be taken with food to minimize abdominal pain and nausea. Other adverse effects include dizziness, somnolence, nervousness and tremor. Uncommonly, cognitive problems including impaired concentration, speech difficulty or confusion have occurred. These effects were uniformly transient and improved with discontinuation of the drug. Nonconvulsive status epilepticus has been reported in patients taking tiagabine (KM Eckardt and BJ Steinhoff, Epilepsia 1998; 39:671; AB Ettinger et al, Epilepsia 1999; 40:1159; T Balslev et al, Europ J Paediatr Neurol 2000; 4:169). No serious or life-threatening adverse effects have been reported.

OXCARBAZEPINE — Oxcarbazepine (*Trileptal* – Medical Letter 2000; 42:33) is chemically similar to carbamazepine but causes less induction of hepatic enzymes. It is approved by the FDA for adjunctive and monotherapy of partial seizures in adults and adjunctive therapy in children more than four years old. Like carbamazepine, oxcarbazepine is also effective in secondarily generalized seizures, but may aggravate myoclonic and absence seizures. Most of the clinical effect is due to the 10-monohydroxy metabolite (MHD), which can be measured in plasma, has a half-life of 8 to 10 hours, and is reduced in concentration in the presence of hepatic enzyme-inducing drugs such as phenobarbital, phenytoin or carbamazepine. Oxcarbazepine is as effective as phenytoin, carbamazepine or valproate in treatment of partial seizures and may be better tolerated. Common adverse effects are somnolence, dizziness, diplopia, ataxia, nausea, vomiting and rash. Cross-reactivity with carbamazepine hypersensitivity occurs in 20% to 30% of patients. Hyponatremia is more common than it is with carbamazepine, and leukopenia can occur, but both are usually not clinically significant. Drug interactions are minor, although oxcarbazepine can increase phenytoin levels and decreases the effectiveness of oral contraceptives. Unlike carbamazepine, oxcarbazepine does not cause induction of its own metabolism (M Bialer et al, Epilepsy Res 2001; 43:11).

LEVETIRACETAM — Levetiracetam (*Keppra* – Medical Letter 2000; 42:33) is used as adjunctive therapy for adults with partial seizures. The mechanism of action in seizure control is unknown. Levetiracetam has no significant drug-drug interactions. The elimination half-life is six to eight hours (M Dooley and GL Plosker, Drugs 2000; 60:871). Common adverse effect are dizziness, somnolence and weakness (JJ Cereghino et al, Neurology 2000; 55:236). No serious or life threatening adverse effects have been reported. Mild decreases in hematocrit and white blood cell count, which do not require discontinuation of drug, occur rarely. Tolerance to the antiepileptic effect of levetiracetam has been reported in animals and anecdotally in people.

ZONISAMIDE — Zonisamide (*Zonegran* – Medical Letter 2000; 42:94) is the most recently approved drug for adjunctive treatment of partial seizures in adults. Despite the limited indication approved by the FDA, it appears to have a broad spectrum of activity (myoclonic seizures, infantile spasms, generalized and atypical absence seizures), and there is considerable experience worldwide with use in children and for other seizure types. Zonisamide is a sulfonamide that, like phenytoin, carbamazepine, and some other anti-seizure drugs, blocks voltage-dependent sodium channels, but it also reduces voltage dependent T-type calcium currents, binds to the GABA receptor and facilitates dopaminergic and serotonergic neurotransmission (CJ Bazil and TA Pedley, Annu Rev Med 1998; 49:135; M Okada et al, Epilepsy Res 1995; 22:193). Zonisamide is a mild carbonic anhydrase inhibitor and has increased the incidence of symptomatic renal stones. It has a long half-life, and may be taken either once or twice daily. Zonisamide is metabolized by CYP3A4. It does not cause induction of hepatic enzymes, and drug interactions are minimal, although 3A4 inducers such as phenytoin and carbamazepine decrease its half-life. Adverse effects, usually transient and self-limited, include somnolence, dizziness, confusion, anorexia, nausea, diarrhea, weight loss and rash (IE Leppik et al, Epilepsy Res 1993; 14:165). Fatal Stevens-Johnson syndrome and toxic epidermal necrolysis have been reported. Oligohydrosis, hyperthermia and heat stroke have occurred in children. Psychosis, aplastic anemia and agranulocytosis have also been reported. Slow titration and dosing with meals may decrease the incidence of adverse effects. Zonisamde is contraindicated in patients allergic to sulfonamides.

DIAZEPAM — Diazepam *(Diastat)* formulated for rectal administration has recently been marketed in the USA for treatment of repetitive seizures. Delivered in this way, diazepam is rapidly and completely absorbed and effective in treating acute repetitive seizures (FE Dreifuss et al, N Engl J Med 1998; 338:1869; JJ Cereghino et al, Neurology 1998; 51:1274). Although not approved for use in status epilepticus, administration of rectal diazepam to children before emergency department treatment decreases the duration of status epilepticus and the incidence of seizure recurrence without serious respiratory depression. *Diastat* is supplied as a prefilled syringe with either pediatric tip (2.5, 5, or 10 mg) or adult tip (10, 15, or 20 mg) for single-dose rectal administration by the patient or caregiver.

ANTICONVULSANTS IN PREGNANCY — Fetal exposure to phenytoin, carbamazepine, valproate, phenobarbital and other older anticonvulsants has been associated with congenital anomalies, including oral cleft, cardiac and neural tube defects, but most pregnant patients exposed to antiepileptic drugs deliver normal infants. High plasma concentrations and use of multiple drugs increase the risk (LB Holmes et al, N Engl J Med 2001; 344:1132). Prophylactic use of folic acid in healthy pregnant women has decreased the incidence of neural tube defects, but has not yet been demonostrated to be protective in women who take antiepileptic drugs during pregnancy (S Hernandez-Diaz et al, N Engl J Med 2000; 343:1608). All women of childbearing age, including those with epilepsy, should take folic acid supplements (MJ Morrell, Neurology 1998; 51 suppl 4:S21). Newer anticonvulsants such as felbamate, gabapentin, lamotrigine, tiagabine and levetiracetam are not teratogenic in animals, but their safety in human pregnancy remains to be established. Topiramate causes limb agenesis in rodents and has been associated with hypospadias in male infants. Zonisamide is also teratogenic in animals. Use of phenytoin, phenobarbital, primidone and carbamazepine can cause hemorrhage in the newborn infant due to vitamin K deficiency, and requires treatment of the mother in the final month of pregnancy and treatment of the newborn.

TREATMENT OF SEIZURES

Seizure Disorder		Drugs	Usual target serum concentrations[1]
PRIMARY GENERALIZED TONIC-CLONIC (GRAND MAL)			
Drugs of Choice:		Valproate[2]	50-120 µg/ml
	OR	Carbamazepine	6-12 µg/ml[3]
	OR	Phenytoin	10-20 µg/ml
Alternatives:		Lamotrigine[6]	3-20 µg/ml
		Topiramate	4-10 µg/ml
		Zonisamide[6]	10-40 µg/ml
		Oxcarbazepine[6]	10-35 µg/ml[7]
		Levetiracetam[6]	5-45 µg/ml
		Primidone	6-12 µg/ml
		Phenobarbital	15-35 µg/ml
PARTIAL, INCLUDING SECONDARILY GENERALIZED			
Drugs of Choice:		Carbamazepine	6-12 µg/ml[3]
	OR	Phenytoin	10-20 µg/ml
	OR	Valproate	50-120 µg/ml
Alternatives:		Lamotrigine	3-20 µg/ml
		Gabapentin[13]	2-16 µg/ml
		Topiramate[13]	4-10 µg/ml
		Tiagabine[13]	100-300 ng/ml
		Zonisamide[13]	10-40 µg/ml
		Oxcarbazepine	10-35 µg/ml
		Levetiracetam[13]	5-45 µg/ml
		Primidone	5-12 µg/ml
		Phenobarbital	15-35 µg/ml

1. Some patients achieve complete seizure control at lower concentrations, and occasional patients need higher concentrations. Serum concentrations may be altered by concurrent use of other drugs.
2. Not FDA-approved unless absence is involved.
3. Monitoring serum concentrations of carbamazepine alone may occasionally be misleading because the assay does not account for an active metabolite, carbamazepine-10,11 epoxide, which contributes to antiepileptic activity and also causes toxic effects. Serum measurements of the active metabolite are available but may be too expensive for routine use.
4. Intolerance to carbamazepine can often be avoided by starting with 100 to 200 mg b.i.d. and increasing the dosage at weekly intervals in increments of 100 to 200 mg per day, up to the usual maintenance dosage.
5. Adjustments in dosage above 300 mg/day for adults should usually be made in 25- or 30-mg increments because metabolism becomes saturated.
6. Not FDA-approved for this indication.

| Total daily dosage | | Usual Dosing |
Adults	Children	Schedule
1000-3000 mg	15-60 mg/kg	bid/tid
800-1600 mg[4]	10-30 mg/kg	bid/tid
300-400 mg[5]	4-8 mg/kg	qd/bid
300-500 mg[8]	5-15 mg/kg[9,10]	bid
200-400 mg[11]	5-9 mg/kg	bid
100-600 mg	Not approved	qd/bid
1200-2400 mg	15-45 mg/kg	bid/tid
1000-3000 mg	Not approved	bid/tid
750-1250 mg[12]	10-25 mg/kg	bid/tid
90-150 mg	2-5 mg/kg	qd/bid
800-1600 mg[4]	10-30 mg/kg	
300-400 mg[5]	4-8 mg/kg	
1000-3000 mg	15-60 mg/kg	
300-500 mg[8]	Not approved	bid
900-2400 mg[14]	25-40 mg/kg[15]	tid
200-400 mg[11]	5-9 mg/kg	bid
32-56 mg[16]	Not approved	tid/qid
100-600 mg	Not approved	qd/bid
1200-2400 mg	15-45 mg/kg	bid/tid
1000-3000 mg	Not approved	bid/tid
750-1250 mg[12]	10-25 mg/kg	bid/tid
90-150 mg	2-5 mg/kg	qd/bid

7. Concentrations of the monohydroxy metabolite (MHD).
8. Dosage is 100 to 500 mg when given with valproate. Dosage for monotherapy is 200 to 500 mg/day.
9. For patients 2 to 12 years old with Lennox-Gastaut syndrome.
10. Dosage is 1 to 5 mg/kg when given with valproate.
11. Start with 25 to 50 mg daily and increase weekly by 25- to 50-mg increments.
12. Start with 50-100 mg daily and increase gradually at two- to three-day intervals.
13. Only FDA approved as adjunct.
14. Start with a dose of 300 mg once or twice daily and increase rapidly up to maintenance dosage.
15. For children more than 5 years old, 25 to 35 mg/kg/day. For children 3 to 4 years old, 40 mg/kg/day.
16. Start with 4 mg daily and increase weekly by 4- to 8-mg increments. Patients taking tiagabine only with a non-enzyme-inducing anticonvulsant (eg. valproate, lamotrigine, gabapentin) may require lower dosage or slower titration.

Seizure Disorder	Drugs	Usual therapeutic serum concentrations[1]
ABSENCE (PETIT MAL)		
Drugs of Choice:	Ethosuximide	40-100 µg/ml
OR	Valproate	50-120 µg/ml
Alternatives:	Lamotrigine[6]	3-20 µg/ml
	Clonazepam	20-80 ng/ml
	Zonisamide[6]	10-40 µg/ml
ATYPICAL ABSENCE, MYOCLONIC, ATONIC		
Drug of Choice:	Valproate[2]	50-120 µg/ml
	Lamotrigine[6]	4-20 µg/ml
Alternatives:	Clonazepam	20-80 ng/ml
	Topiramate[6]	4-10 µg/ml
	Zonisamide[6]	10-40 µg/ml
	Felbamate[13]	30-100 µg/ml

| Total daily dosage | | Usual Dosing |
Adults	Children	Schedule
750-1250 mg	20-40 mg/kg	bid
1000-3000 mg	15-60 mg/kg	bid/tid
300-500 mg	Not approved	bid
1.5-20 mg	0.05-0.2 mg/kg	bid/tid
100-600 mg	Not approved	qd/bid
1000-3000 mg	15-60 mg/kg	bid/tid
300-500 mg[8]	5-15 mg/kg[9,10]	bid
1.5-20 mg	0.05-0.2 mg/kg	bid/tid
200-400 mg[11]	Not approved	bid
100-600 mg	Not approved	qd/bid
2400-3600 mg	15-60 mg/kg	bid/tid/qid

COST OF SOME ANTIEPILEPTIC DRUGS

Drug	Usual adult daily dosage	Cost*
Carbamazepine – average generic price	800 to 1600 mg	$ 28.80
Tegretol (Novartis)		58.80
Tegretol XR (Novartis)		57.60
Carbatrol (Shire Richwood)		64.80
Clonazepam – average generic price	1.5 to 20 mg	45.00
Klonopin (Roche Labs)		73.80
Ethosuximide – *Zarontin* (Pfizer)	750 to 1250 mg	81.00
Felbamate – *Felbatol* (Wallace)	2400 to 3600 mg	162.50
Gabapentin – *Neurontin* (Pfizer)	900 to 3600 mg	101.70
Lamotrigine – *Lamictal* (GlaxoSmithKline)	300 to 500 mg	135.60
Levetiracetam – *Keppra* (UCB Pharma)	1000 to 3000 mg	100.20
Oxcarbazepine – *Trilepta* (Novartis)	1200 to 2400 mg	175.20
Phenobarbital – average generic price	90 to 150 mg	6.30
Phenytoin – average generic price	300 to 400 mg	12.60
Dilantin Kapseals (Pfizer)		25.20
Primidone – average generic price (HCFA)	750 to 1250 mg	38.70
Mysoline (Wyeth-Ayerst)		88.20
Tiagabine – *Gabitril* (Abbott)	32 to 56 mg	158.40
Topiramate – *Topamax* (McNeil)	200 to 400 mg	175.20
Valproate	1000 to 3000 mg	
Valproic acid – low generic price (HCFA)		46.80
Depakene (Abbott)		192.00
Divalproex sodium – *Depakote* (Abbott)		94.80
Depakote ER (Abbott)		97.80
Zonisamide – *Zonegran* (Elan Pharma)	100 to 600 mg	51.90

* Average cost to the patient for a 30-day supply with lowest recommended dosage, based on data from retail pharmacies nationwide, provided by Scott-Levin's *Source*™ *Prescription Audit (SPA)*, May 2000 to April 2001.

DRUGS FOR CHRONIC HEART FAILURE

The choice of drugs for treatment of heart failure continues to evolve. In recent years it has become increasingly recognized that drugs used in heart failure produce beneficial effects through neurohormonal as well as hemodynamic mechanisms (M Packer and JN Cohn et al, Am J Cardiol 1999; 83 suppl 2A:9A).

ACE INHIBITORS — Angiotensin-converting enzyme (ACE) inhibitors improve symptoms in patients with heart failure, sometimes within days, but more commonly with a delay of 4 to 12 weeks. In sufficient doses, these drugs slow the progression of heart failure and prolong survival in patients with impaired left ventricular function (MD Flather et al, Lancet 2000; 355:1575). An analysis of data from two controlled trials in about 2000 patients with left ventricular dysfunction (SOLVD) found that enalapril (*Vasotec*, and others), compared to placebo, significantly reduced the risk of hospitalization for heart failure in white patients but not in blacks (DV Exner et al, N Engl J Med 2001; 344:1351). A double-blind randomized trial (ATLAS) in more than 3000 patients with class II-IV congestive heart failure compared high doses (32.5 or 35 mg daily) with low doses (2.5 or 5 mg daily) of lisinopril (*Prinivil, Zestril*), but participating physicians were permitted to add a second ACE inhibitor at their discretion. The results indicated, according to the investigators, that patients with heart failure should not be maintained on very low doses of an ACE inhibitor, and that the difference in efficacy between intermediate and high doses is likely to be very small (M Packer et al, Circulation 1999; 100:2312).

Adverse Effects – The most common adverse effects of ACE inhibitors are related to suppression of angiotensin II (hypotension and renal insufficiency) and increases in concentrations of endogenous kinins (cough and angioedema). Those related to angiotensin II suppression can be ameliorated by decreasing the dose of diuretic taken concurrently. Those related to kinins can be relieved by replacing the ACE inhibitor with one of the angiotensin II receptor blockers, which do not increase kinins.

ANGIOTENSIN RECEPTOR BLOCKERS — Whether angiotensin II receptor antagonists such as losartan *(Cozaar)*, valsartan *(Diovan)*, irbesartan *(Avapro)*, candesartan (*Atacand*) or telmisartan *(Micardis)* are as effective as ACE inhibitors in heart failure has not been established by clinical trials. In a double-blind study of more than 3000 patients with class II-IV heart failure (ELITE II), all-cause mortality was lower with captopril (*Capoten*, and others) than with losartan, although the difference was not statistically significant (B Pitt et al, Lancet 2000; 355:1582). Another study found that the addition of valsartan to ACE inhibitors and other drugs led to a reduction in hospitalization but not in mortality; in the subset of patients already taking a beta-blocker as well as an ACE inhibitor, however, no benefit was detectable when valsartan was added, and there was a trend toward increased morbidity and mortality (JN Cohn et al, VaL-HeFT Trial, Presented at AHA Scientific Sessions, 2000).

BETA-BLOCKERS — Even though short-term use of beta-blockers can decrease the contractility of the heart, blocking the effects of sympathetic activation can produce long-term clinical benefits in patients with heart failure whether or not coronary heart disease is the cause. Controlled trials have shown that metoprolol (*Lopressor, Toprol XL*, and others), bisoprolol *(Zebeta)* or carvedilol *(Coreg)* added to other drugs improve ejection fraction, slow the progression of heart failure and decrease the risk of death and frequency of hospitalization in patients with mild to moderate (class II-III) heart failure (Medical Letter 2000; 42:54).

An analysis of four trials in more than 1000 patients with class II-IV heart failure found that carvedilol, which has both beta- and alpha-adrenergic blocking properties, lowered the risk of death or hospitalization from any cause by 48% in black patients and by 30% in nonblacks, and reduced the risk of worsening heart failure by 54% in blacks and 57% in nonblacks (CW Yancy et al, N Engl J Med 2001; 344:1385). Carvedilol also has decreased mortality after myocardial infarction in patients with left ventricular dysfunction with or without heart failure (The CAPRICORN Investigators, Lancet

2001; 357:1358). Recently, COPERNICUS, a randomized placebo-controlled trial of carvedilol in heart failure patients with symptoms at rest or on minimal exertion, was stopped early because of a 35% reduction in mortality with carvedilol; patients with significant fluid retention and those receiving positive inotropic drugs were excluded from this study (M Packer et al, N Engl J Med 2001; 344:1651). An ongoing clinical trial (COMET) in patients with heart failure is comparing carvedilol with metoprolol.

Dosage and Adverse Effects – Beta-blockers should be started with a low dose; hypotension and worsening failure may occur during the first two to four weeks of treatment. These drugs should only be given to patients already taking optimal doses of a diuretic and an ACE inhibitor, especially in class IV heart failure. They should not be given to patients who have shown signs of clinical instability in the previous week. Dosage should be increased gradually over several weeks; full clinical benefits may not occur for one to three months.

DIURETICS — Most patients with heart failure have fluid retention. In these patients, diuretics relieve symptoms of heart failure, but do not slow progression of the underlying disease, and their effect on survival is unknown (E Lonn, BMJ 2000; 320:1188). Diuretics that act on the loop of Henle, such as furosemide (*Lasix*, and others), bumetanide (*Bumex*, and others) or torsemide (*Demadex*), are more effective than thiazide diuretics, such as chlorothiazide (*Diuril*, and others), which act on the distal tubule. Patients resistant to an oral diuretic may respond to intravenous administration or to concurrent use of two diuretics with different sites of action.

Adverse Effects – The most common adverse effect of diuretic therapy is hypokalemia, which can be decreased or prevented by taking oral potassium supplements or by concurrent use of an ACE inhibitor and/or a potassium-sparing diuretic such as spironolactone (*Aldactone*, and others), amiloride (*Midamor*, and others) or triamterene (*Dyrenium*).

DIGITALIS — Digoxin (*Lanoxin*, and others) can decrease the symptoms of heart failure, increase exercise tolerance and decrease the frequency of hospitalization. The results of a large long-term study indicate that adding digoxin to other drugs decreases the rate of hospitalization, especially among the sickest patients, but does not affect survival (The Digitalis Investigation Group, N Engl J Med 1997; 336:525).

Dosage and Adverse Effects – The optimal dosage of digoxin is not clear. Clinical studies have often used a daily dosage of 0.25 to 0.50 mg, but many clinicians prescribe 0.125 to 0.25 mg daily. In trials demonstrating benefit from digoxin, the mean digoxin dose was 0.38 mg/day, corresponding to a mean serum digoxin level of 1.2 ng/ml. The most common adverse effects of digitalis glycosides are conduction disturbances, cardiac arrhythmias, nausea, vomiting, confusion and visual disturbances.

VASODILATORS — Concurrent use of two vasodilators, hydralazine and isosorbide dinitrate, can produce sustained improvement in left ventricular ejection fraction. In patients with mild to moderate heart failure already taking digitalis and diuretics, the combination improved exercise tolerance and had a beneficial effect on mortality, but less than that of enalapril (JN Cohn et al, V-HEFT II, N Engl J Med 1991; 325:303). Hydralazine/isosorbide dinitrate has been reported to be particularly effective in black patients (P Carson et al, J Cardiac Fail 1999; 5:178). No data are available on use of the hydralazine-nitrate combination in patients also taking an ACE inhibitor or beta-blocker. Hydralazine/isosorbide dinitrate frequently causes headache; gastrointestinal disturbances, palpitations and nasal congestion can occur.

SPIRONOLACTONE — One double-blind, placebo-controlled trial in more than 1,600 patients with severe heart failure found that adding the aldosterone-receptor inhibitor spironolactone (*Aldactone*, and others) to standard treatment led to a 30% decrease in total mortality and a 35% reduction in hospitalization for heart failure. Hyperkalemia was rare, even in patients also taking an ACE inhibitor (B Pitt et al, RALES, N Engl J Med 1999; 341:709)

Most adverse effects of spironolactone with recommended dosages for heart failure (12.5 to 50 mg) are mild and respond to withdrawal of the drug. Hyperkalemia can occur, especially in patients taking potassium supplements or an ACE inhibitor, and in those with renal impairment. Spironolactone has antiandrogenic activity, and can cause painful gynecomastia, menstrual irregularities and impotence.

CONCLUSION — Unless there is a specific contraindication, all patients with heart failure due to left ventricular dysfunction should take both an ACE inhibitor and a beta-blocker. Angiotensin II receptor blockers have not been shown to be as effective as ACE inhibitors for treatment of heart failure; in patients who cannot tolerate ACE inhibitors because of cough or angioedema, they are appropriate second-line agents. A combination of hydralazine and isosorbide dinitrate may also be a useful second-line treatment. Digoxin can decrease symptoms and lower the rate of hospitalization for heart failure, but does not decrease total mortality. Diuretics relieve congestive symptoms due to volume overload. Addition of spironolactone to conventional therapy appears to decrease mortality in patients with severe heart failure, but can cause hyperkalemia.

DRUGS FOR HYPERTENSION

Drugs available in the USA for treatment of chronic hypertension, their dosages and adverse effects are listed in the table below and discussed in the text beginning on page 110. Drugs for treatment of hypertensive emergencies are not discussed here.

SOME ORAL ANTIHYPERTENSIVE DRUGS

Drug and daily maintenance dosage	Cost[1]	Frequent or severe adverse effects*
ANGIOTENSIN-CONVERTING ENZYME (ACE) INHIBITORS		
Benazepril – 10-80 mg in 1 or 2 doses		
Lotensin (Novartis)	$26.40	
Captopril – 12.5-150 mg in 2 or 3 doses		Cough; hypotension, particu-
average generic price	8.10[2]	larly with diuretic use or
Capoten (Apothecon)	27.90[2]	volume depletion; rash; acute
Enalapril – 2.5-40 mg in 1-2 doses		renal failure with bilateral re-
average generic price	20.70	nal artery stenosis or stenosis
Vasotec (Merck)	26.40	of the artery to a solitary kid-
Fosinopril – 10-40 mg in 1 or 2 doses		ney; angioedema; hyper-
Monopril (Bristol-Myers Squibb)	28.50	kalemia if also taking potassi-
Lisinopril – 5-40 mg in 1 dose		um supplements or potas-
Prinivil (Merck)	27.60	sium-sparing diuretics; mild-
Zestril (AstraZeneca)	27.60	to-moderate loss of taste;
Moexipril – 7.5-30 mg in 1 or 2 doses		hepatotoxicity; pancreatitis;
Univasc (Schwarz)	21.00	blood dyscrasias and renal
Perindopril – 4-8 mg in 1 or 2 doses		damage rare except in pa-
Aceon (Solvay)	30.90	tients with renal dysfunction;
Quinapril – 5-80 mg in 1 or 2 doses		increased fetal mortality with
Accupril (Parke-Davis)	30.60	second- and third-trimester
Ramipril – 1.25-20 mg in 1 or 2 doses		exposure; may decrease ex-
Altace (Monarch)	25.80	cretion of lithium
Trandolapril – 1-4 mg in 1 dose		
Mavik (Knoll)	23.70	

* In addition to the adverse effects listed, antihypertensive drugs may interact adversely with other drugs taken at the same time (*Medical Letter Handbook of Adverse Drug Interactions*, 2001).

1. Average cost to the patient for 30 days' treatment with the lowest dose tablet or capsule, based on data from retail pharmacies nationwide provided by Scott-Levin's *Source*™ *Prescription Audit* (SPA), December 1999-November 2000.

2. Cost based on purchase of 30 of the smallest tablet size available.

Drug and daily maintenance dosage	Cost[1]	Frequent or severe adverse effects*
ANGIOTENSIN II RECEPTOR ANTAGONISTS		
Candesartan cilexetil – 8-32 mg in 1 dose		
Atacand (AstraZeneca)	$37.80	
Eprosartan – 400-800 mg in 1 or 2 doses		
Teveten (Unimed)	28.80	
Irbesartan – 150-300 mg in 1 dose		Similar to ACE inhibitors, but
Avapro (Bristol-Myers Squibb)	38.40	do not cause cough and rare-
Losartan – 25-100 mg in 1 or 2 doses		ly cause angioedema, loss of
Cozaar (Merck)	38.10	taste or hepatic dysfunction
Telmisartan – 40-80 mg in 1 dose		
Micardis (Abbott)	39.90	
Valsartan – 80-320 mg in 1 dose		
Diovan (Novartis)	38.10	
BETA-ADRENERGIC BLOCKING DRUGS		
Atenolol – 25-100 mg in 1 or 2 doses		
average generic price	$ 8.70	
Tenormin (AstraZeneca)	32.40	
Betaxolol – 5-40 mg in 1 dose		
average generic price	24.60[2]	Fatigue; depression; brady-
Kerlone (Searle)	28.80[2]	cardia; impotence; decreased
Bisoprolol – 5-20 mg in 1 dose		exercise tolerance; congestive
average generic price	36.30	heart failure; worsening of
Zebeta (ESI Lederle)	37.80	peripheral arterial insuffi-
Metoprolol – 50-200 mg in 1 or 2 doses		ciency; may aggravate allergic
average generic price	7.80	reactions; bronchospasm;
Lopressor (Novartis)	21.90	may mask symptoms of and
extended release – 50-400 mg in 1 dose		delay recovery from
Toprol-XL (AstraZeneca)	19.50	hypoglycemia; Raynaud's
Nadolol – 20-320 mg in 1 dose		phenomenon; insomnia; vivid
average generic price	18.30	dreams or hallucinations;
Corgard (Apothecon)	41.10	acute mental disorder; in-
Propranolol – 40-240 mg in 2 doses		creased serum triglycerides,
average generic price	8.40	decreased HDL cholesterol;
Inderal (Wyeth-Ayerst)	17.10	sudden withdrawal may lead
extended release – 60-240 mg in 1 dose		to exacerbation of angina and
average generic price	27.60	myocardial infarction
Inderal-LA (Wyeth-Ayerst)	33.90	
Timolol – 10-40 mg in 2 doses		
average generic price	16.20	
Blocadren (Merck)	31.80	

---

* In addition to the adverse effects listed, antihypertensive drugs may interact adversely with other drugs taken at the same time (*Medical Letter Handbook of Adverse Drug Interactions*, 2001).

Drug and daily maintenance dosage	Cost[1]	Frequent or severe adverse effects*

BETA-BLOCKERS WITH INTRINSIC SYMPATHOMIMETIC ACTIVITY

Acebutolol – 200-1200 mg in 1 or 2 doses		Similar to other beta-adrener-
average generic price	$21.30	gic blocking drugs, but with
Sectral (Wyeth-Ayerst)	37.50	less resting bradycardia and
Carteolol – 2.5-10 mg in 1 dose		lipid changes; acebutolol has
Cartrol (Abbott)	35.70	been associated with a posi-
Penbutolol – 20 mg in 1 dose		tive antinuclear antibody test
Levatol (Schwarz)	42.90	and occasional drug-induced
Pindolol – 10-60 mg in 2 doses		lupus
average generic price	21.60	
Visken (Novartis)	63.00	

BETA-BLOCKERS WITH ALPHA-1 BLOCKING ACTIVITY

Carvedilol – 12.5-50 mg in 2 doses		Similar to other beta-
Coreg (GlaxoSmithKline)	$92.40	adrenergic blocking drugs,
Labetalol – 200-1200 mg in 2 doses		but more orthostatic hypoten-
average generic price	24.60	sion; hepatotoxicity with la-
Normodyne (Key)	34.80	betalol
Trandate (GlaxoSmithKline)	34.80	

DIURETICS

THIAZIDE-TYPE (Usually once daily)[3]

Chlorothiazide – 125-500 mg		
average generic price	$ 5.40[2]	
Diuril (Merck)	6.60[2]	Hyperuricemia; hypokalemia;
Hydrochlorothiazide – 12.5-50 mg		hypomagnesemia; hypergly-
average generic price	14.10	cemia; hyponatremia; hyper-
Esidrix (Novartis)	6.90[2]	calcemia; hypercholesterole-
Microzide (Watson)	16.50	mia; hypertriglyceridemia;
Chlorthalidone – 12.5-50 mg		pancreatitis; rashes and other
average generic price	5.40[2]	allergic reactions; sexual dys-
Indapamide – 1.25-5 mg		function; photosensitivity
average generic price	12.30	reactions; may decrease ex-
Lozol (Aventis)	28.80	cretion of lithium
Metolazone –		
Zaroxolyn (Medeva) – 1.25-5 mg	22.80[2]	
Mykrox (Medeva) – 0.5-1 mg	27.60	

1. Average cost to the patient for 30 days' treatment with the lowest dose tablet or capsule, based on data from retail pharmacies nationwide provided by Scott-Levin's *Source*™ *Prescription Audit* (SPA), December 1999-November 2000.

2. Cost based on purchase of 30 of the smallest tablet size available.

3. Other available thiazide-type diuretics include: bendroflumethiazide *(Naturetin)*, hydroflumethiazide *(Diucardin)*, methyclothiazide (*Enduron*, and others), polythiazide *(Renese)* and trichlormethiazide *(Naqua*, and others).

Drug and daily maintenance dosage	Cost[1]	Frequent or severe adverse effects*
LOOP		
Bumetanide – 0.5-5 mg in 2 or 3 doses	$ 8.70[2]	Dehydration; circulatory collapse; hypokalemia; hyponatremia; hypomag-nesemia; hyperglycemia; metabolic alkalosis; hyperuricemia; blood dyscrasias; rashes; lipid changes as with thia-zide-type diuretics
average generic price		
Bumex (Roche)	12.00[2]	
Ethacrynic acid – 25-100 mg in 2 or 3 doses		
Edecrin (Merck)	12.30	
Furosemide – 20-320 mg in 2 or 3 doses		
average generic price	4.50[2]	
Lasix (Aventis)	7.80[2]	
Torsemide – 5-20 mg in 1 or 2 doses		
Demadex (Roche)	18.00	
POTASSIUM-SPARING		
Amiloride – 5-10 mg in 1 or 2 doses		Hyperkalemia; GI distur-bances; rash; headache
average generic price	13.80	
Midamor (Merck)	16.80	
Spironolactone – 12.5-100 mg in 1 or 2 doses		Hyperkalemia; hypona-tremia; mastodynia; gynecomastia; menstrual abnormalities; GI distur-bances; rash
average generic price	9.30[2]	
Aldactone (Pharmacia)	15.90[2]	
Triamterene – 50-150 mg in 1 or 2 doses		Hyperkalemia; GI distur-bances; nephrolithiasis
Dyrenium (GlaxoSmithKline)	26.40	
CALCIUM-CHANNEL BLOCKERS		
Diltiazem – extended-release 120-360 mg in 2 doses		
average generic price	$40.20	
Cardizem SR (Biovail)	57.00	
extended-release (once per day)		
average generic price	30.30	
Cardizem CD (Biovail) – 120-360 mg in 1 dose	37.80	
Dilacor XR (Watson) – 120-480 mg in 1 dose	32.70	Dizziness; headache; ede-ma; constipation (espe-cially verapamil); AV block; bradycardia; heart failure; lupus-like rash with diltiazem
Diltia XT (Andrx) – 120-480 mg in 1 dose	22.80	
Tiazac (Forest) – 120-480 mg in 1 dose	30.90	
Verapamil – 120-480 mg in 2 or 3 doses		
average generic price	21.60	
Calan (Searle)	39.60	
extended-release – 120-480 mg in 1 or 2 doses		
average generic price (tablets)	24.00	
Calan SR (Searle)	33.90	
Covera-HS (Pharmacia) – 180-480 mg in 1 dose	37.50	
average generic price (capsules)	31.80	

Drug and daily maintenance dosage	Cost[1]	Frequent or severe adverse effects*
Isoptin SR (Knoll)	$34.20	
Verelan (Wyeth-Ayerst) – 120-480 mg in 1 dose	44.40	
DIHYDROPYRIDINES		
Amlodipine – 2.5-10 mg in 1 dose		
Norvasc (Pfizer)	39.90	
Felodipine – 2.5-10 mg in 1 dose		
Plendil (AstraZeneca)	31.50	
Isradipine– 5-10 mg in 2 doses		
DynaCirc (Novartis)	46.20	
extended-release – 5-10 mg in 1 dose		Dizziness; headache; peri-
DynaCirc CR	39.00	pheral edema (more than
Nicardipine – 60-120 mg in 3 doses		with verapamil and dil-
average generic price	32.40	tiazem; more common in
Cardene (Roche)	42.30	women); flushing;
extended-release – 60-120 mg in 2 doses		tachycardia; rash; gin-
Cardene SR (Roche)	43.80	gival hyperplasia
Nifedipine – extended release 30-90 mg in 1 dose		
average generic price	36.90	
Adalat CC (Bayer)	35.70	
Procardia XL (Pfizer)	41.10	
Nisoldipine – 10-60 mg in 1 dose		
Sular (AstraZeneca)	30.30	
ALPHA-ADRENERGIC BLOCKERS		
Prazosin – First day: 1 mg at bedtime	$ 5.40[2]	Syncope with first dose
Maintenance: 1-20 mg in 2 or 3 doses		(less likely with terazosin
average generic price		and doxazosin); dizziness
Minipress (Pfizer)	15.00[2]	and vertigo; headache;
		palpitations; fluid reten-
		tion; drowsiness; weak-
		ness; anticholinergic
		effects; priapism
Terazosin – First day: 1 mg at bedtime		
Maintenance: 1-20 mg in 1 dose		
average generic price	41.10	
Hytrin (Abbott)	53.70	
Doxazosin – First day: 1 mg at bedtime		
Maintenance: 1-16 mg in 1 dose		
average generic price	24.90	
Cardura (Pfizer)	30.90	

Drug and daily maintenance dosage	Cost[1]	Frequent or severe adverse effects*
CENTRAL ALPHA-ADRENERGIC AGONISTS		
Clonidine – 0.1-0.6 mg in 2 or 3 doses		CNS reactions similar to
average generic price	$ 5.70[2]	methyldopa, but more seda-
Catapres (Boehringer Ingelheim)	22.20[2]	tion and dry mouth; brady-
transdermal – one patch weekly		cardia; heart block; rebound
(0.1 to 0.3 mg/day)		hypertension (less likely with patch); contact dermatitis from patch
Catapres TTS (Boehringer Ingelheim)	39.88	
Guanabenz – 4-64 mg in 2 doses		Similar to clonidine
average generic price	15.60[2]	
Wytensin (Wyeth-Ayerst)	27.00[2]	
Guanfacine – 1-3 mg in 1 dose		Similar to clonidine, but milder
average generic price	21.10	
Tenex (Robins)	67.80	
Methyldopa – 250 mg-2 grams in 2 doses		Drowsiness; sedation; fatigue;
average generic price	13.80	depression; dry mouth;
Aldomet (Merck)	19.80	orthostatic hypotension; bradycardia; heart block; colitis; hepatitis; hepatic necrosis; Coombs' positive hemolytic anemia; lupus-like syndrome; thrombocytopenia; red cell aplasia; impotence
DIRECT VASODILATORS		
Hydralazine – 40-200 mg in 2-4 doses		Tachycardia; aggravation of
average generic price	$ 8.40	angina; headache; dizziness; fluid retention; nasal congestion; lupus-like syndrome; hepatitis
Minoxidil – 2.5-40 mg in 1 or 2 doses		Tachycardia; aggravation of
average generic price	1.20	angina; marked fluid retention; pericardial effusion; hair growth on face and body
Loniten (Pharmacia)	20.70	

Drug and daily maintenance dosage	Cost[1]	Frequent or severe adverse effects*
PERIPHERAL ADRENERGIC NEURON ANTAGONISTS		
Guanadrel – 10-75 mg in 2 doses *Hylorel* (Medeva)	$47.70[2]	Orthostatic hypotension; exercise hypotension; bradycardia, sodium and water retention; retrograde ejaculation; occasional diarrhea
Reserpine – 0.05-0.1 mg in 1 dose average generic price	9.90[2]	Nasal stuffiness; drowsiness; GI disturbances; bradycardia; psychic depression, nightmares with high doses; tardive dyskinesia

ANGIOTENSIN-CONVERTING ENZYME (ACE) INHIBITORS — ACE inhibitors are effective and well tolerated for treatment of hypertension. They are less effective in black patients unless combined with a thiazide diuretic. ACE inhibitors do not affect plasma lipids or glucose tolerance. They have been shown to reduce mortality in patients with coronary artery disease (The Heart Outcomes Prevention Evaluation Study Investigators [HOPE], N Engl J Med 2000; 342:145), prolong survival in patients with heart failure or left ventricular dysfunction after a myocardial infarction, and preserve renal function in patients with diabetes. They may also preserve renal function in patients with non-diabetic nephropathies. ACE inhibitors and beta-adrenergic blocking drugs appear to be superior to calcium-channel blockers in preventing progression to renal failure in black patients with hypertensive nephropathy (African American Study of Kidney Disease and Hypertension, presented at the Annual Meeting of the American Society of Nephrology, October 2000).

ANGIOTENSIN II RECEPTOR ANTAGONISTS — **Losartan, valsartan, irbesartan, candesartan, telmisartan** and **eprosartan** (Medical Letter 1999; 41:105), drugs that interfere with binding of angiotensin II to AT_1 receptors, are effective in lowering blood pressure without causing cough. Whether angiotensin II receptor antagonists provide the same cardiac and renal protection as ACE inhibitors remains to be established. In one large trial comparing losartan to captopril in patients with heart failure, all-cause mortality was lower with captopril, but the difference was not statistically significant (B Pitt et al [ELITE II], Lancet

2000; 355:1582). Like ACE inhibitors, these drugs may be less effective in black patients and should not be used during pregnancy.

BETA-ADRENERGIC BLOCKING DRUGS — Beta-blockers are effective for treatment of hypertension, but like ACE inhibitors, may be less effective in black patients. A beta-blocker alone appears to be less effective than a diuretic alone for treatment of the elderly.

Propranolol, timolol, nadolol, pindolol, penbutolol, and **carteolol** are "nonselective" beta-blockers; in low doses **bisoprolol, atenolol, metoprolol, acebutolol** and **betaxolol** are "cardioselective," with a greater effect on cardiac (beta$_1$) adrenergic receptors than on beta$_2$-adrenergic receptors in bronchi and blood vessels. These drugs become less selective as dosage is increased, and even low doses may cause bronchospasm. **Pindolol, acebutolol, penbutolol,** and **carteolol** have intrinsic sympathomimetic activity (ISA) and unlike other beta-blockers generally do not increase serum triglyceride concentrations or decrease HDL cholesterol. Beta-blockers with ISA can lower blood pressure with less decrease in heart rate at rest and may be preferred for patients who develop symptomatic bradycardia or postural hypotension with other beta-blockers. Beta-blockers without ISA are preferred in patients with angina or a history of myocardial infarction.

Labetalol combines nonselective beta-blockade and minimal ISA with alpha-adrenergic receptor blockade. It decreases blood pressure more promptly than other beta-blockers, is equally effective in black and white patients, and does not affect serum lipids. **Carvedilol** is also both an alpha- and a nonselective beta-blocker, but has no ISA. It has been promoted more for treatment of heart failure than for treatment of hypertension (Medical Letter 1999; 41:13).

DIURETICS — Diuretics have been shown to decrease mortality in patients with hypertension. Thiazide diuretics have been shown to reduce the incidence of stroke and cardiovascular events in elderly patients with isolated systolic hypertension (SHEP Cooperative Research Group, JAMA 1991; 265:3255). Many **thiazide-type diuretics** are used to treat hypertension; **hydrochlorothiazide** and **chlorthalidone** are the most widely used. **Metolazone** and **indapamide** may be effective in patients with impaired renal function when thiazides are not. Many patients, particularly older ones, can be treated with small doses of diuretics equivalent to 12.5 mg to 25 mg of hydrochlorothiazide once daily. Doses as low as 6.25 mg are now used to enhance the effectiveness of other drugs while minimizing adverse effects such as hypokalemia. **Loop diuretics** can be used to treat hypertension in patients with renal insufficiency (creatinine clearance below 30 to 50 ml/min). In patients without renal insufficiency, they may be less effective than thiazides for treatment of hypertension.

Potassium-sparing diuretics are used with other diuretics to prevent or correct hypokalemia. These drugs can cause hyperkalemia, particularly in patients with renal impairment and those taking other drugs that decrease aldosterone secretion, such as ACE inhibitors and angiotensin II receptor antagonists. The aldosterone receptor antagonist spironolactone has been shown to reduce mortality in ACE inhibitor-treated patients with congestive heart failure who are also taking digoxin and loop diuretics (B Pitt et al, N Engl J Med 1999; 341:709).

CALCIUM-CHANNEL BLOCKERS — The calcium-channel blockers cause vasodilatation, which decreases peripheral resistance. The cardiac response to decreased vascular resistance is variable; with some dihydropyridines (**felodipine, nicardipine, nisoldipine** and immediate-release **nifedipine**), an initial reflex increase in heart rate usually occurs, but **isradipine, verapamil, diltiazem**, sustained-release **nifedipine** and **amlodipine** cause little or no change in heart rate. Verapamil and diltiazem slow heart rate, can affect atrioventricular (AV) conduction and should be used with caution in patients also taking a beta-blocker. Short-acting calcium-channel blockers, particularly nifedipine, should not be used for treatment of hypertension (Medical Letter 1997; 39:13). Two recent meta-analyses have suggested that the risk of coronary artery disease and heart failure might be higher in patients treated with calcium-channel blockers compared to those treated with ACE inhibitors, beta-blockers and diuretics (Blood Pressure Lowering Treatment Trialists' Collaboration, Lancet 2000; 355:1955; M Pahor et al, Lancet 2000; 355:1949). In patients with diabetes, use of a calcium channel blocker has been associated with an increased risk of myocardial infarction compared to use of an ACE inhibitor (RO Estacio et al, N Engl J Med 1998; 338:645).

CENTRAL ALPHA-ADRENERGIC AGONISTS — Drugs such as **clonidine, guanabenz, guanfacine** and **methyldopa** do not inhibit reflex responses as completely as sympatholytic drugs that act peripherally, but frequently cause sedation, dry mouth and depression.

ALPHA-ADRENERGIC BLOCKING DRUGS — **Prazosin**, **terazosin** and **doxazosin** cause less tachycardia than direct vasodilators (hydralazine, minoxidil) but more frequent postural hypotension, particularly following the first dose. Treatment of essential hypertension with doxazosin has been associated with an increased incidence of heart failure compared to treatment with a diuretic. It is unknown whether this will occur with prazosin or terazosin (ALLHAT Collaborative Research Group, JAMA 2000; 283:1967). Alpha-blockers may provide symptomatic relief from prostatism in men, but may cause stress incontinence in women, and have a higher incidence of postural hypotension in elderly patients.

DIRECT VASODILATORS — Direct vasodilators frequently produce reflex tachycardia, but rarely cause orthostatic hypotension. They should usually be given with a beta-blocker or a centrally-acting drug to minimize the reflex increase in heart rate and cardiac output, and with a loop diuretic to avoid sodium and water retention. They should be avoided in patients with coronary artery disease. **Hydralazine** maintenance dosage should be limited to 200 mg per day to decrease the possibility of a lupus-like reaction. **Minoxidil**, a potent drug that rarely fails to lower blood pressure, should be reserved for severe hypertension refractory to other drugs. Minoxidil usually causes hirsutism and can cause severe fluid retention.

PERIPHERAL ADRENERGIC NEURON ANTAGONISTS — These drugs can cause troublesome adverse effects and are rarely used. **Reserpine** is an effective antihypertensive (HS Fraser, Clin Pharmacol Ther 1996; 60:368), but in doses higher than currently recommended, it can cause severe depression. **Guanadrel** usually decreases cardiac output and may lower systolic pressure more than diastolic; postural and exertional hypotension occur commonly and are aggravated by vasodilatation caused by heat, exercise or alcohol.

COMBINATION PRODUCTS — Combination products are convenient and can improve compliance, but in general are not recommended for initial therapy.

CHOICE OF DRUGS — The best tolerated drugs for treatment of hypertension are diuretics (particularly in low doses) and angiotensin II receptor antagonists. Beta-adrenergic blockers, ACE inhibitors and calcium-channel blockers generally have mild adverse effects. Diuretics alone and together with beta-blockers have been shown in large-scale clinical trials to decrease mortality in patients with hypertension (JNC VI, Arch Intern Med 1997; 157:2413). Some Medical Letter consultants believe calcium-channel blockers should be reserved for patients who do not respond to or cannot tolerate diuretics, beta-blockers, ACE inhibitors or angiotensin II receptor antagonists.

In special categories of patients, one type of drug may offer advantages. ACE inhibitors should be considered in patients with **diabetes**, particularly with nephropathy, and in those with **heart failure** or **left ventricular dysfunction**. A beta-blocker may be the best choice for hypertensive patients with **angina pectoris** or **migraine**, for those who have had a **myocardial infarction** and for some patients with **heart failure**. For patients with **hyperlipidemia**, an ACE inhibitor, alpha-blocker or calcium-channel blocker might be a good choice. Diuretics and calcium-channel blockers are more effective than beta-blockers, ACE inhibitors or angiotensin II receptor antagonists in **black patients**. A diuretic with or without a beta-blocker, or a long-acting dihydropyridine calcium-channel blocker, is preferred in **older patients** with isolated systolic hypertension.

Even when drugs are carefully chosen to fit individual needs, patients' responses may vary. Generally, if the first drug chosen is ineffective or poorly tolerated, a drug from another class should be substituted. If more than one drug is necessary and a diuretic was not used initially, most Medical Letter consultants would add a diuretic.

SOME COMBINATION PRODUCTS

Drug	Cost*
DIURETIC COMBINATIONS	
Hydrochlorothiazide 25 or 50 mg/spironolactone 25 or 50 mg	
average generic price	$9.90
Aldactazide (Pharmacia)	17.10
Hydrochlorothiazide 25 or 50 mg/triamterene 37.5 or 75 mg	
average generic price	11.40
Dyazide (GlaxoSmithKline)	15.00
Maxzide (Bertek)	17.40
Hydrochlorothiazide 50 mg/amiloride 5 mg	
Moduretic (Merck)	19.80
BETA-ADRENERGIC BLOCKERS AND DIURETICS	
Atenolol 50 or 100 mg/chlorthalidone 25 mg	
average generic price	15.00
Tenoretic (AstraZeneca)	38.40
Bisoprolol 2.5, 5 or 10 mg/hydrochlorothiazide 6.25 mg	
average generic price	29.40
Ziac (Lederle)	36.60
Metoprolol 50 or 100 mg/hydrochlorothiazide 25 or 50 mg	
Lopressor HCT (Novartis)	26.10
Propranolol 40 or 80 mg/hydrochlorothiazide 25 mg	
average generic price	9.00
Inderide (Wyeth-Ayerst)	36.60
Propranolol extended-release 80, 120 or 160 mg/hydrochlorothiazide 50 mg	
Inderide LA (Wyeth-Ayerst)	51.30
Timolol 10 mg/hydrochlorothiazide 25 mg	
Timolide (Merck)	23.70
ACE INHIBITORS AND DIURETICS	
Benazepril 5, 10, 20 mg/hydrochlorothiazide 6.25, 12.5 or 25 mg	
Lotensin HCT (Novartis)	26.70
Captopril 25 or 50 mg/hydrochlorothiazide 15 or 25 mg	
average generic price	15.60
Capozide (Apothecon)	31.20
Enalapril 5 or 10 mg/hydrochlorothiazide 12.5 or 25 mg	
Vaseretic (Merck)	35.10

* Average cost to the patient for 30 days' treatment with the lowest dose tablet or capsule once per day, based on data from retail pharmacies nationwide provided by Scott-Levin's *Source™ Prescription Audit* (SPA), December 1999-November 2000.

Drug	Cost*
ACE Inhibitors and Diuretics *(continued)*	
Fosinopril 10 or 20 mg/hydrochlorothiazide 12.5 mg	
Monopril HCT (Bristol-Myers Squibb)	$29.40
Lisinopril 10 or 20 mg/hydrochlorothiazide 12.5 or 25 mg	
Prinzide (Merck)	31.50
Zestoretic (AstraZeneca)	31.80
Moexipril 7.5 or 15 mg/hydrochlorothiazide 12.5 or 25 mg	
Uniretic (Schwarz)	23.70
Quinipril 10 or 20 mg/hydrochlorothiazide 12.5 or 25 mg	
Accuretic (Parke Davis)	31.50
ANGIOTENSIN II RECEPTOR ANTAGONISTS AND DIURETICS	
Candesartan 16 or 32 mg/hydrochlorothiazide 12.5 mg	
Atacand HCT (AstraZeneca)	52.20
Irbesartan 150 or 300 mg/hydrochlorothiazide 12.5 mg	
Avalide (Bristol-Myers Squibb)	47.10
Losartan 50 or 100 mg/hydrochlorothiazide 12.5 or 25 mg	
Hyzaar (Merck)	38.10
Telmisartan 40 or 80 mg/hydrochlorothiazide 12.5 mg	
Micardis HCT (Abbott)	42.92**
Valsartan 80 or 160 mg/hydrochlorothiazide 12.5 mg	
Diovan HCT (Novartis)	41.40
CALCIUM-CHANNEL BLOCKERS AND ACE INHIBITORS	
Amlodipine 2.5 or 5 mg/benazepril 10 or 20 mg	
Lotrel (Novartis)	51.00
Felodipine 2.5 or 5 mg/enalapril 5 mg	
Lexxel (AstraZeneca)	39.30
Verapamil extended-release 180 or 240 mg/trandolapril 1, 2 or 4 mg	
Tarka (Knoll)	45.60
OTHER COMBINATIONS	
Hydralazine 25 or 50 mg/hydrochlorothiazide 25 or 50 mg	
average generic price	7.20
Methyldopa 250 or 500 mg/hydrochlorothiazide 15, 25, 30 or 50 mg	
average generic price	7.80
Aldoril (Merck)	17.40
Clonidine 0.1, 0.2 or 0.3 mg/chlorthalidone 15 mg	
Combipres (Boehringer Ingelheim)	22.80

* Average cost to the patient for 30 days' treatment with the lowest dose tablet or capsule once per day, based on data from retail pharmacies nationwide provided by Scott-Levin's *Source*™ *Prescription Audit* (SPA), December 1999-November 2000.

** Cost based on AWP listings in *Drug Topics Red Book Update*, June 2001.

HYPNOTIC DRUGS

Many drugs are used to treat insomnia, but for some patients nonpharmacological treatments such as changing sleep habits, relaxation training and cognitive therapy may be more effective than drugs (J Wagner et al, Ann Pharmacother 1998; 32:680; CM Morin et al, JAMA 1999; 281:991).

NONPRESCRIPTION HYPNOTICS — Two **antihistamines**—diphenhydramine (*Nytol, Benadryl* and others) and doxylamine (*Unisom*, and others)—are currently approved by the FDA for sale as "sleep-aids" without a prescription. They can cause daytime sedation, impairment of performance skills such as driving, and troublesome anticholinergic effects such as dry mouth and urinary retention. **Alcohol** causes initial CNS depression followed by rebound excitation, disrupting sleep. **Melatonin** has shown some promise, but adequate controlled trials are lacking, and the purity, hypnotic dose and adverse effects of melatonin products have not been established (D Avery et al, Ann Med 1998; 30:122; J Pepping, Am J Health Syst Pharm 1999; 56:2520). **Valerian root** is a mild hypnotic that may improve the quality of sleep and appears to have few adverse effects, but as with other herbal products, optimal dosage is unclear and purity is a concern (SL Plushner, Am J Health Syst Pharm 2000; 57:328).

OLDER PRESCRIPTION HYPNOTICS — **Chloral hydrate** (*Noctec*, and others) is an effective hypnotic when used for a few nights to treat transient insomnia. Within two weeks, however, its effectiveness can wane, and continued use often leads to physical dependence. Withdrawal of the drug can cause disrupted sleep and intense nightmares. The usual hypnotic dose of chloral hydrate is 0.5 to 1 gram; fatalities have occurred following ingestion of as little as 4 grams. **Barbiturates** have the disadvantages of a narrow therapeutic ratio, lethality in overdosage, rapid development of tolerance, high liability for physical dependence and abuse, and many drug interactions (*The Medical Letter Handbook of Adverse Drug Interactions*, 2001, page 130). **Ethchlorvynol** (*Placidyl*, and others), which also has been associated with dependence and abuse, has some serious adverse effects and can be lethal in overdosage.

BENZODIAZEPINE RECEPTOR AGONISTS — Benzodiazepines decrease the time to onset of sleep (sleep latency), prolong the first two stages of sleep, and suppress stages 3 and 4 (deep sleep) and REM sleep. Although all benzodiazepines have hypnotic activity, only triazolam, estazolam, temazepam, flurazepam and quazepam are labeled for use as hypnotics in the USA. Zaleplon and zolpidem, which are not benzodiazepines but bind selectively to benzodiazepine receptors, decrease sleep latency with little effect on sleep stages. Zaleplon is a rapid-acting hypnotic that is less potent and has a shorter duration of action than zolpidem. Zaleplon does not decrease premature awakenings or increase total sleep time, but appears to have a low risk of next-day residual effects, even with middle-of-the-night use (Medical Letter 1996; 38:60; 1999; 41:93; M Dooley and GL Plosker, Drugs 2000; 60:413).

Adverse Effects – Fatal overdosage is rare with any oral benzodiazepine receptor agonist unless it is taken with alcohol or other central-nervous-system depressants. The effectiveness of these drugs as hypnotics can persist for weeks or even several months, but all probably can produce physical dependence, especially with higher doses and longer duration of treatment. All benzodiazepine agonists can cause anterograde amnesia and psychiatric effects. Those with a short duration of action may be the most likely to cause daytime anxiety and rebound insomnia. Drugs with a long duration of action may cause daytime sedation and motor impairment. Benzodiazepines with an intermediate duration of action theoretically could avoid both rebound and hangover effects, but both can occur with these drugs as well (MM Mitler, Sleep 2000; 23 suppl 1:S39). Use of benzodiazepines in elderly patients has been associated with an increased incidence of falls and hip fractures, and impairment of memory (RM Leipzig et al, J Am Geriat Soc 1999; 47:30; JT Hanlon et al, Clin Pharmacol Ther 1998; 64:684). Some Medical Letter consultants believe that zolpidem and zaleplon will prove safer than older, longer-acting benzodiazepines, but direct comparisons are lacking.

SOME BENZODIAZEPINE RECEPTOR AGONISTS
USED TO TREAT INSOMNIA

Drug	Duration	Onset of action	Hypnotic dose	Dose in Elderly	Cost[1]
Zaleplon[2] – *Sonata* (Wyeth-Ayerst)	ultra-short	rapid 15-30 min	10-20 mg	5 mg	$15.47
Zolpidem[2] – *Ambien* (Searle)	short	rapid 30 min	10 mg	5 mg	15.75
Triazolam – average generic price *Halcion* (Pharmacia)	short	rapid 15-30 min	0.125-0.25 mg	0.125 mg	4.13 7.63
Oxazepam[3] – average generic price	short to intermediate	intermediate to slow 45-60 min	15-30 mg	10-15 mg	4.27
Estazolam – average generic price *ProSom* (Abbott)	intermediate	rapid to intermediate 15-60 min	1-2 mg	0.5-1 mg	5.81 8.89
Lorazepam[3] – average generic price *Ativan* (Wyeth-Ayerst)	intermediate	intermediate 30-60 min	1-2 mg	0.25-1 mg	4.41 7.56
Temazepam – average generic price *Restoril* (Novartis)	intermediate	intermediate to slow 45-60 min	15-30 mg	7.5-15 mg	3.01 7.14
Clonazepam[3] – average generic price *Klonopin* (Roche)	long	intermediate 30-60 min	0.5 mg	0.25 mg	3.43 5.74
Diazepam[3] – average generic price *Valium* (Roche)	long	rapid 15-30 min	5-10 mg	2.5-5 mg	1.26 6.16
Flurazepam – average generic price *Dalmane* (Roche)	long	intermediate 30-60 min	30 mg	7.5 mg	2.24 11.20
Quazepam – *Doral* (Wallace)	long	intermediate 20-45 min	15 mg	7.5 mg	19.32

1. Average cost to the patient for 7 doses at the lowest recommended hypnotic dosage, based on data from retail pharmacies nationwide provided by Scott-Levin's *Source*™ *Prescription Audit (SPA)*, June 2000 to May 2001.
2. Not a benzodiazepine, but binds to benzodiazepine receptors.
3. Insomnia is not an FDA-approved indication.

ANTIDEPRESSANTS — Trazodone (*Desyrel*, and others) a non-tricyclic, non-SSRI antidepressant, has been used effectively in a single 25- to 150-mg dose at bedtime to relieve insomnia in depressed and non-depressed patients, including some taking a selective serotonin reuptake inhibitor (SSRI) or bupropion (*Wellbutrin*, and others). Orthostatic hypotension can occur, and male patients should be warned about the rare occurrence of priapism. Nefazodone *(Serzone)* and mirtazapine *(Remeron)* have also been used in a single dose at bedtime to produce somnolence (ME Thase, J Clin Psychiatry 1999; 60 suppl 17:28).

CONCLUSION — All drugs available for treatment of insomnia have some drawbacks, especially with prolonged use. Short-term use of a short-acting benzodiazepine receptor agonist is generally effective and safe, but may not prevent early morning awakening. For patients with this problem, a benzodiazepine with an intermediate duration of action may be more helpful.

CHOICE OF LIPID-REGULATING DRUGS

New recommendations for drug treatment of hypercholesterolemia, if widely followed, will lead to a marked increase in the number of people taking lipid-regulating drugs (Expert Panel on Detection, Evaluation and Treatment of High Blood Cholesterol in Adults, JAMA 2001; 285:2486). Drugs that lower serum concentrations of low-density lipoprotein (LDL) cholesterol can prevent formation, slow progression and cause regression of atherosclerotic lesions, improve vasodilation and decrease mortality. These drugs must be continued indefinitely; when they are stopped, plasma cholesterol concentrations generally return to pretreatment levels. Other plasma lipids and lipoproteins also play a role in the pathogenesis of atherosclerosis, but their importance in prevention and treatment of vascular disease is less well defined.

LIPOPROTEINS, TRIGLYCERIDES AND APOLIPOPROTEINS — Most of the cholesterol in plasma and in atherosclerotic lesions is normally in **low-density lipoprotein (LDL) cholesterol**; high plasma concentrations of LDL are associated with an increased risk of atherosclerotic cardiovascular disease. Besides total plasma LDL concentration, the size and density of LDL particles may affect risk; small denser forms appear to be more atherogenic.

A low plasma concentration of **high-density lipoprotein (HDL) cholesterol** is a strong risk factor for coronary heart disease, even when LDL and total plasma cholesterol are normal. Trials of lipid-regulating drugs have shown an association between increases in HDL cholesterol and reduction in clinical coronary events, but more evidence is needed.

Triglycerides in plasma are carried mainly in chylomicrons and in very-low-density lipoproteins (VLDL) and intermediate-density lipoproteins (IDL) (RJ Havel, Curr Opin Lipidol, 2000; 11:615). Although hypertriglyceridemia is associated with increased cardiovascular risk, it is not clear whether lowering elevated triglyceride levels decreases cardiovascular events.

Apolipoproteins are protein constituents of lipoproteins. High concentrations of apolipoprotein B (the major structural protein of LDL, IDL and VLDL) and of lipoprotein(a) have been associated with an increased risk of coronary heart disease (SH Wild et al, Arterioscler Thromb Vasc Biol 1997; 17:239). High concentrations of apolipoprotein A1 are associated with high levels of HDL cholesterol and a lower risk of coronary disease.

HMG-CoA REDUCTASE INHIBITORS (STATINS) — HMG-CoA reductase inhibitors, often called "statins", inhibit the enzyme that catalyzes the rate-limiting step in cholesterol synthesis. They are more effective than other drugs in lowering plasma concentrations of LDL cholesterol. They also may increase HDL cholesterol (by up to about 15% with high doses) and reduce levels of triglycerides.

HMG-CoA REDUCTASE INHIBITORS (STATINS)

Drugs	FDA-Approved Daily Dosage*	Usual Decrease in LDL Cholesterol	Cost[1]
Atorvastatin – *Lipitor* (Pfizer)	Initial: 10 mg once Maximum: 80 mg once	35%-40% 50%-60%	$57.30 98.40
Cerivastatin – *Baycol* (Bayer)	Initial: 0.4 mg once Maximum: 0.8 mg once	34%-38% 42%-44%	45.90 68.40
Fluvastatin – *Lescol* (Novartis) extended-release – *Lescol XL*	Initial: 20 mg once Maximum: 40 mg bid[1] 80 mg once	20%-25% 30%-35% 35%-38%	41.40 82.80 55.20
Lovastatin – *Mevacor* (Merck)	Initial: 20 mg once Maximum: 80 mg once[2]	25%-30% 35%-40%	69.60 247.80
Pravastatin – *Pravachol* (Bristol-Myers Squibb)	Initial: 20 mg once Maximum: 40 mg once	25%-32% 30%-35%	69.60 112.50
Simvastatin – *Zocor* (Merck)	Initial: 20 mg once Maximum: 80 mg once	35%-40% 45%-50%	112.20 113.10

* For initial treatment of patients with only modest elevations of LDL or a history of poor tolerance for these drugs, some Medical Letter consultants use lower doses.

1. Average cost to the patient for 30 days' treatment based on data from retail pharmacies nationwide provided by Scott-Levin's *Source*™ *Prescription Audit* (SPA) May 2000 to April 2001.

2. Or divided b.i.d.

Effect on Coronary Disease – Three large trials in patients with **clinical coronary artery disease** have shown that treatment with simvastatin or pravastatin can reduce mortality from all causes, lower cardiac mortality and morbidity, and reduce the incidence of stroke in patients with high or even average initial cholesterol levels (Scandinavian Simvastatin Survival Study Group, Lancet 1994; 344:1383; FM Sacks et al, N Engl J Med 1996; 335:1001; LIPID Study Group, N Engl J Med 1998; 339:1349). A placebo-controlled trial of atorvastatin 80 mg/day started within 96 hours after hospital admission for myocardial infarction was associated with a lower incidence of ischemic events in the subsequent 16 weeks, but the large number of patients lost to follow-up in the atorvastatin group calls the results into question (GG Schwartz et al [MIRACL], JAMA 2001; 285:1711).

For **prevention**, pravastatin in hypercholesterolemic men without a previous myocardial infarction, and lovastatin in patients with average total but below-average HDL cholesterol without previous coronary disease, reduced the risk of subsequent coronary events (J Shepherd et al [WOSCOP], N Engl J Med 1995; 333:1301; JR Downs et al [AFCAPS/TexCAPs], JAMA 1998; 279:1615).

Non-Cardiovascular Effects – Both lovastatin and simvastatin have marked osteogenic effects in rodents (G Mundy et al, Science 1999; 286:1946). Some observational studies have suggested that statin treatment reduces fracture risk in elderly patients (KA Chan et al, Lancet 2000; 355:2185; CR Meier et al, JAMA 2000; 283:3205; PS Wang et al, JAMA 2000; 283:3211), but others have offered no support for this hypothesis (IC Reid et al, Lancet 2001; 357:509; T-P van Staa et al, JAMA 2001; 285:1850). Analysis of data from a primary prevention study in hypercholesterolemic men suggests that pravastatin may prevent or delay development of type II diabetes (DJ Freeman et al, Circulation 2001; 103:357).

Adverse Effects – Statins are generally better tolerated than other lipid-regulating drugs; some patients who cannot tolerate one statin may tolerate another. Mild, transient gastrointestinal disturbances and muscle pain can occur. Severe myalgia and muscle weakness, with or without increased serum creatinine phosphokinase, have been reported. Rarely, severe rhabdomyolysis and myoglobinuria leading to renal failure have occurred. The risk and severity of myopathy may be increased in patients with hepatic dysfunction, renal failure (especially with pravastatin), serious infections, hypothyroidism or advanced age.

An increase in plasma aminotransferase activities to more than three times normal occurs in 1% to 2% of patients taking higher doses of these drugs, but symptomatic hepatitis has been rare. The risk of hepatic toxicity is increased in patients who abuse alcohol. A recent report suggests that patients who develop hepatitis with one statin may subsequently be able to tolerate another (A Nakad et al, Lancet 1999; 353:1763).

Fatigue and loss of a sense of well being can occur, particularly with high doses of statins, according to Medical Letter consultants. Impotence has been reported with simvastatin (IW Boyd, Ann Pharmacother 1996; 30:1199; G Jackson, BMJ 1997; 315:31). Some patients have associated statins with sleep disturbances.

In one of two large secondary prevention studies using 40 mg pravastatin daily, 12 women out of 286 actively treated developed breast cancer, compared to one among the 290 placebo-treated women (SJ Lewis et al, J Am Coll Cardiol 1998; 32:140). The other trial, in which 756 women received pravastatin, showed no increase in the incidence of breast cancer after six years of treatment (LIPID Study Group, N Engl J Med 1998; 339:1349). With up to seven years' follow-up in controlled trials, patients treated with lovastatin, pravastatin and simvastatin have had no detectable increase in the overall incidence of cancer.

Drug Interactions – Statin-induced myopathy is often caused by drug interactions. Lovastatin and simvastatin undergo extensive first-pass metabolism in the liver by CYP3A4, and their serum concentrations can be increased dramatically by concurrent use of CYP3A4 inhibitors such as itraconazole *(Sporanox)*, ketoconazole *(Nizoral)*, erythromycin, clarithromycin *(Biaxin)*, cyclosporine *(Sandimmune*, and others), nefazodone *(Serzone)* and many HIV protease inhibitors. Grapefruit juice inhibits intestinal (but not hepatic) CYP3A4 and may increase serum concentrations of lovastatin and simvastatin; drinking a small amount of juice in the morning and taking the statin in the evening should minimize the interaction (DG Bailey, Br J Clin Pharmacol 1998; 46:101; JD Rogers, Clin Pharmacol Ther 1999; 66:358). Atorvastatin and cerivastatin are also metabolized at least partly by CYP3A4, but 3A4 inhibitors produce only modest increases in their serum concentrations. Gemfibrozil also decreases metabolism of lovastatin, simvastatin and cerivastatin; rhabdomyolysis has occurred with concurrent use. Pravastatin is metabolized by sulfation, not by the cytochrome system, and is the least affected by other drugs, but gemfibrozil or cyclosporine taken concurrently can increase serum levels of pravastatin and increase the risk of myopathy. Fluvastatin is mainly metabolized by CYP2C9; few interactions have been reported. Concurrent use of lovastatin, simvastatin or fluvastatin with oral anticoagulants has increased the hypoprothrombinemic effect (*The Medical Letter Handbook of Adverse Drug Interactions*, 2001, page 69).

FIBRIC ACID DERIVATIVES ("FIBRATES") — Gemfibrozil (*Lopid*, and others), fenofibrate *(Tricor)*, bezafibrate (*Bezalip* – not available in the USA) and clofibrate (*Atromid-S*, and others) are used mainly to lower triglycerides and to increase HDL cholesterol. They may lower LDL cholesterol, but when they decrease elevated triglycerides, LDL cholesterol may increase in some patients. Fibrates shift the size distribution of LDL to larger, more buoyant particles that may be less atherogenic than smaller, denser forms. While drugs that mainly lower LDL (statins and bile-acid sequestrants) show a linear relationship between the degree of cholesterol lowering and the reduction in clinical coronary events, fibrates show a much greater reduction in clinical events than predicted from the degree of cholesterol lowering. This suggests that the effect of fibrates on coronary disease is mediated by a different mechanism, possibly associated with their effects on triglycerides and HDL cholesterol (GR Thompson and PJ Barter, Curr Opin Lipidol 1999; 10:521). No fibrate trial, however, has ever shown significant reduction in total mortality.

Fibrates may potentiate the effects of oral anticoagulants and oral hypoglycemic agents. They may also interact with statins to increase the risk of rhabdomyolysis (*The Medical Letter Handbook of Adverse Drug Interactions*, 2001, pages 203, 277 and 288). Cholelithiasis, hepatitis and myositis can occur.

Gemfibrozil – A large, placebo-controlled primary prevention trial in hypercholesterolemic men showed that patients treated with gemfibrozil had a statistically significantly lower number of myocardial infarctions, but not of deaths from all causes. Gemfibrozil caused gastrointestinal symptoms, and both cholecystectomies and appendectomies were more frequent in gemfibrozil-treated patients (MH Frick et al, N Engl J Med 1987; 317:1237).

A large, placebo-controlled trial in men with coronary heart disease and low HDL cholesterol (mean 32 mg/dl), low LDL cholesterol (mean 112 mg/dl) and moderate triglycerides (mean 160 mg/dl) showed that after five years the incidence of death from coronary heart disease, nonfatal myocardial infarction or stroke was statistically significantly lower with gemfibrozil, even though LDL cholesterol values were unaffected. The incidence of stroke was reduced by 25% (6.0% to 4.6%), which was not statistically significant, but transient ischemic attacks and carotid endarterectomies were reduced by 59% and 65%, respectively. The rate of death from all causes was reduced by 11% (17.4% to 15.7%), which was not statistically significant (HB Rubins et al [VA-HIT], N Engl J Med 1999; 341:410). Increases in HDL concentrations were associated with a lower incidence of coronary events (SJ Robins et al, JAMA 2001; 285:1585). A subset analysis showed that virtually all of the clinical benefit occurred in patients with diabetes or hyperinsulinemia (SJ Robins et al, Circulation 2000; 102:II-847).

Fenofibrate – Taken once daily with a meal, fenofibrate (*Tricor* – Medical Letter 1998; 40:68) may be more effective than gemfibrozil in lowering serum LDL cholesterol and triglyceride concentrations. A placebo-controlled trial in about 400 diet-treated type II diabetic patients with angiographic evidence of coronary artery disease and average plasma lipid concentrations showed that fenofibrate, after more than three years, had slowed the rate of progression of coronary disease by 40% on angiography, and reduced the risk of coronary clinical events from 50% to 38%, which was not statistically significant (DAIS Investigators, Lancet 2001; 357:905).

Bezafibrate – Bezafibrate, available in Europe and Canada, or a placebo was given for five years to diet-treated men with hyperlipidemia and a history of premature myocardial infarction. Active treatment lowered triglycerides (31%) and increased HDL cholesterol (9%) without affecting LDL cholesterol concentrations. Both the progression of coronary atherosclerosis and clinical coronary events were significantly reduced (C-G Ericsson et al, Lancet 1996; 347:849). In a large placebo-controlled trial in patients with stable angina or a previous myocardial infarction who had average plasma lipid concentrations, bezafibrate did not reduce the incidence of myocardial infarction and death significantly after six years. A contributing cause of the negative outcome may have been that many placebo-treated patients received other lipid-lowering drugs during the last years of the trial (The BIP Study Group, Circulation 2000; 102:21).

Clofibrate – Because of its toxicity (a high mortality rate due to malignant and gastrointestinal disease in some early studies), the use of clofibrate should be limited to patients with severe hypertriglyceridemia unresponsive to other fibrates, niacin, or a combination of niacin and fibrate.

NIACIN (NICOTINIC ACID) — Niacin, which inhibits production of very-low-density lipoprotein (VLDL) particles in the liver, increases HDL cholesterol more than any other drug. It also decreases triglycerides, remnant lipoproteins, lipoprotein(a), and total plasma and LDL cholesterol, changing LDL particles from small and dense to large and buoyant forms (JR Guyton et al, Arch Intern Med 2000; 160:1177). Lower doses (1500 to 2000 mg/day) can affect triglycerides and HDL cholesterol markedly; higher doses may be required for substantial reductions of LDL cholesterol. In one placebo-controlled trial, men with one or more previous myocardial infarctions who took niacin had a lower incidence of nonfatal myocardial reinfarctions and, nine years later, a lower mortality rate (PL Canner et al, J Am Coll Cardiol 1986; 8:1245).

Adverse Effects – Niacin can cause skin flushing and pruritus, gastrointestinal distress, blurred vision, fatigue, glucose intolerance, hyperuricemia, hepatic toxicity, exacerbation of peptic ulcer and, rarely, dry eyes or hyperpigmentation. Starting with a low dose and pretreatment with aspirin (325 mg) or ibuprofen (200 mg) can diminish cutaneous reactions. Hepatic toxicity, sometimes severe, has been reported mainly with older sustained-release preparations, especially at doses higher than 2000 mg/d (JM McKenney et al, JAMA 1994; 271:672). *Niaspan* appears to be better tolerated.

BILE-ACID SEQUESTRANTS — The resins cholestyramine (*Questran*, and others) and colestipol *(Colestid)*, and the hydrophilic polymer colesevelam hydrochloride (*Welchol* – Medical Letter 2000; 42:102), which are not absorbed from the gastrointestinal tract, can lower serum concentrations of LDL cholesterol by up to 20%. These drugs also tend to increase HDL cholesterol and, in patients with hypertriglyceridemia, cholestyramine, colestipol and, to a lesser extent, colesevelam raise plasma triglycerides. A seven-year primary prevention study in hypercholesterolemic men showed that cholestyramine reduced the incidence of non-fatal myocardial infarction and death from coronary heart disease compared to placebo (The Lipid Research Clinics Primary Prevention Trial, JAMA 1984; 251:351).

Adverse Effects – The adverse effects of colestipol and cholestyramine are similar; constipation occurs frequently and may be accompanied by heartburn, nausea, eructation and bloating, but these symptoms may disappear over time. Giving the drugs in moderate doses (8 to 10 grams daily or less) just before meals improves tolerance (but decreases effectiveness), and increased dietary fiber or a fiber supplement, such as psyllium (*Metamucil* and others), may relieve constipation and bloating. There appear to be fewer reports of gastrointestinal adverse effects and interference with absorption of other drugs with colesevelam than with cholestyramine or colestipol (*The Medical Letter Handbook of Adverse Drug Interactions* 2001, pages 195 and 211), and statins maintain their cholesterol-lowering effect when taken at the same time as colesevelam.

COST OF SOME OTHER LIPID-REGULATING DRUGS

Drug	Daily dosage	Cost*
Bile-Acid Sequestrants		
Cholestyramine granules –	8-12 grams resin bid	
average generic price		$21.60
Locholest granules (Warner Chilcott)		34.80
Questran granules (Apothecon)		27.60
Cholestyramine Light packets –	8-12 grams resin bid	
average generic price		30.00
Questran Light granules		46.80
Prevalite packets (Upsher-Smith)		67.20
Colestipol – *Colestid* granules (Pharmacia)	10-15 grams, bid	50.40
Colestid tablets	10 grams, divided	135.00
Colesevelam – *Welchol* (Sankyo Pharma)	3.8 grams once or 1.9 grams bid	133.20
Fibrates		
Clofibrate – average generic price	1 gram bid	81.60
Atromid S (Wyeth-Ayerst)		134.40
Gemfibrozil – average generic price	600 mg bid	28.80
Lopid (Pfizer)		84.60
Fenofibrate – *Tricor* (Abbott)	200 mg once	70.50
Niacin**		
immediate-release – average generic price	1 gram tid	12.60
Niacor (Upsher-Smith)		48.60
extended-release – average generic price	2 grams once	10.80
Niaspan (Kos)		65.40

* Cost to the patient for 30 days' treatment with the lowest recommended dosage based on data from retail pharmacies nationwide provided by Scott-Levin's *Source*™ *Prescription Audit* (SPA) May 2000 to April 2001.

** Some niacin products are available over the counter.

FISH OIL — Long-chain, highly unsaturated omega-3 fatty acids (present in cold-water fish and commercially available in capsules) can decrease triglycerides and may lower lipoprotein(a) after long-term intake (SM Marcovina et al, Arterioscler Thromb Vasc Biol 1999; 19:1250). They have little effect on LDL cholesterol, but may increase HDL. A large, randomized, open-label study of survivors after a recent acute myocardial infarction compared the effect of 1 g daily of omega-3 fatty acids with that of no supplements. After three years, the incidence of the combined endpoint (death, nonfatal myocardial infarction and stroke) was 14.6% in the control group compared to 12.3% in those treated with fish oil, which was statistically significant (GISSI-Prevenzione Investigators, Lancet 1999; 354:447). Omega-3 fatty acids can interfere with platelet function and possibly cause bleeding.

COMBINATIONS — When tolerable doses of a single drug do not lower blood lipids sufficiently, two or more drugs can be used together. In patients with hypercholesterolemia, concurrent use of a statin with a bile-acid sequestrant or niacin, or with both, can effectively lower LDL cholesterol. Combining a statin with niacin can simultaneously lower LDL and raise HDL cholesterol. In severe hypertriglyceridemia not adequately controlled by diet and a single drug, combining niacin with a fibrate, and possibly even with fish oil, may substantially lower triglycerides. For combined hypercholesterolemia and hypertriglyceridemia, concurrent use of a statin with either niacin or a fibrate can be useful, but both niacin and gemfibrozil increase the risk of statin-induced myopathy.

CONCLUSION — HMG-CoA reductase inhibitors ("statins") are the lipid-regulating drugs of first choice for treatment of most patients at risk for coronary heart disease. A long-term decrease in the rate of mortality or major coronary events has been documented with pravastatin, simvastatin and lovastatin. Maximum doses of atorvastatin decrease LDL cholesterol the most. When both LDL and HDL cholesterol are low in patients at risk for coronary heart disease, gemfibrozil has been shown to lower the incidence of coronary events.

DRUGS FOR MIGRAINE

Drugs for treatment of migraine are listed in the table below. All are most effective when taken before the pain becomes severe. Some drugs for prevention of migraine are listed in the table on page 137. Treatment of migraine in the emergency room, which may involve use of intravenous drugs, is not included here.

SOME DRUGS FOR TREATMENT OF MIGRAINE ATTACK

Drug	Dosage[1]	Cost[2]
Ergot Alkaloids		
Dihydroergotamine		
D.H.E. 45 (Novartis)	1 mg IM or SC; can be repeated twice at 1-hour intervals (max. 3 mg/attack, 6 mg/week)	$15.36[3]
Migranal Nasal Spray (Novartis)	One spray (0.5 mg) into each nostril, repeated 15 minutes later (2 mg/dose; max. 3 mg/24 hours)	19.67[3]
Ergotamine *Ergomar* (Lotus Biochemical)	2-mg sublingual tablet, can be repeated q30 min. x 2 PRN (max. 3 tabs/attack)	5.02
Ergotamine 1 mg/caffeine 100 mg *Cafergot* (Novartis)	2 tablets orally, then 1 q30min. x 4 PRN (max. 6 tabs/attack)	2.18
Ergotamine 2 mg/caffeine 100 mg *Cafergot* (Novartis)	One rectal suppository; can be repeated once 1 hour later	5.39
5-HT$_1$ Receptor Agonists ("Triptans")		
Naratriptan – *Amerge* (GlaxoSmithKline)	1- or 2.5-mg tablet, can be repeated 4 hours later (max. 5 mg/24 hours)	16.59

1. Recommended by the manufacturer.
2. Average cost to the patient for treating one migraine attack using lowest recommended dosage based on data from retail pharmacies nationwide provided by Scott Levin's *Source*™ *Prescription Audit (SPA)*, May 2000 to April 2001.
3. Price based on AWP listings in *Drug Topics Red Book* 2001 and June *Update*.

Drug	Dosage[1]	Cost[2]
Rizatriptan – *Maxalt, Maxalt MLT* (Merck)	5- or 10-mg tablet or wafer; can be repeated in 2 hours (max. 30 mg/24 hours)[4]	$14.45 14.31
Sumatriptan – *Imitrex* (GlaxoSmithKline)	6 mg SC; can be repeated in 1 hour (max. 2 injections/24 hours)[5]	48.15
	25, 50 or 100 mg orally[6]; can be repeated in 2 hours (max. 200 mg/24 hours)	15.39
	5 or 20 mg intranasally; can be repeated after 2 hours (max. 40 mg/24 hours)	21.85[4]
Zolmitriptan – *Zomig, Zomig ZMT* (AstraZeneca)	2.5 or 5 mg orally; can be repeated in 2 hours (max. 10 mg/24 hours)	13.56 13.89
Opioid Analgesics		
Butorphanol – *Stadol NS* (Bristol-Myers Squibb)	One spray in one nostril; can be repeated in the other nostril in 60-90 minutes; the same sequence can be repeated 3 to 5 hours after the second dose	5.57-10.46[4,7]

4. Patients taking propranolol should only use the 5-mg tablet or wafer (max. 15 mg/24 hours).
5. Preferably in the lateral thigh or deltoid. A second dose is not usually effective if pain does not respond to the first, but is recommended for treatment of a recurrent migraine attack.
6. The recommended oral dose of sumatriptan is 25, 50 or 100 mg in the USA; in Europe and Canada it is 50 or 100 mg. Some data suggest that 100 mg may not provide greater relief than 50 mg, except in mild attacks.
7. Each 2.5-ml bottle contains 25 mg of butorphanol. After initial priming each bottle delivers 14 to 15 1-mg doses, depending on frequency of use. With intermittent use requiring repriming before each dose, the 2.5-ml bottle will deliver 8 to 10 doses.

ANALGESICS — Treatment with an analgesic may be sufficient for mild or moderate forms of migraine. **Aspirin** can be effective; it is widely used for treatment of migraine both alone and in combinations such as *Fiorinal*, which contains caffeine and butalbital. **Acetaminophen** has been used for migraine both alone (RB Lipton et al, Arch Intern Med 2000; 160:3486) and in combinations such as *Fioricet* or *Esgic*, which also contain caffeine and butalbital, and *Midrin*, which contains isometheptene (a sympathomimetic amine) and dichloralphenazone (a chloral hydrate compound). A combination of acetaminophen with aspirin and caffeine (*Excedrin*

Migraine) has been approved by the FDA for over-the-counter use in migraine. Ibuprofen *(Advil Migraine, Motrin Migraine)* is also FDA-approved for OTC treatment of migraine attacks. Other nonsteroidal anti-inflammatory drugs (NSAIDs) such as naproxen sodium *(Anaprox,* and others) have been effective in relieving the pain of some migraine attacks. Decreased gastric motility during an acute migraine attack may interfere with absorption of analgesics, and overuse (more than two or three days a week) can cause an increase in headache frequency (drug-induced rebound headache). Metoclopramide *(Reglan,* and others) taken promptly at the onset of symptoms can enhance absorption of other oral drugs by increasing gastric motility and prevent the nausea associated with many migraine attacks.

Oral opioid combinations and injected opioids are effective for relief of pain, but they produce the usual opioid adverse effects, and frequent use can lead to drug dependence. **Butorphanol** nasal spray *(Stadol NS)*, an opioid agonist-antagonist, has been effective for relief of moderate to severe migraine, but drug dependence and abuse have been reported.

ERGOT ALKALOIDS — **Ergotamine** tartrate, a non-specific serotonin agonist and a vasoconstrictor, has been used for many years for treatment of moderate to severe migraine headache. When used more than two days a week, it can cause drug-induced rebound headache. Ergotamine is available alone in sublingual tablets and combined with caffeine in oral tablets and suppositories. Nausea and vomiting are fairly common with ergotamine, but can be prevented by pretreatment or concurrent use of an antiemetic, such as prochlorperazine *(Compazine,* and others). Serious adverse effects, such as vascular (including coronary) occlusion and gangrene, are rare, but can occur with overdosage (more than 6 mg in 24 hours or 10 mg per week). These effects may be potentiated by triptans, beta-adrenergic blockers, dopamine *(Intropin,* and others), or CYP3A4 inhibitors such as erythromycin *(The Medical Letter Handbook of Adverse Drug Interactions,* 2001, page 270). Liver disease or fever can accelerate symptoms of ergotism.

Dihydroergotamine, which can be injected subcutaneously, intramuscularly or intravenously, or sprayed intranasally, is also effective in treating migraine attacks unresponsive to analgesics. It is a weaker arterial vasoconstrictor than ergotamine and causes fewer adverse effects; it can cause diarrhea and muscle cramps, but rebound headache apparently does not occur. Dihydroergotamine nasal spray *(Migranal)* relieves migraine after two hours in about 50% of patients and after four hours in up to 70%, with a 15% incidence of headache recurrence within 24 hours.

5-HT$_1$ RECEPTOR AGONISTS ("TRIPTANS") — **Sumatriptan** *(Imitrex)* has been marketed in the USA in a formulation for subcutaneous self-injection, in an oral formulation, and as a nasal spray. A selective serotonin-receptor agonist with a short duration of action, it appears to be more effective than ergotamine for treatment of acute migraine attacks. The injection and nasal spray formulations often begin to produce relief in 10 to 15 minutes, compared to one to two hours with the tablets. A subcutaneous injection of sumatriptan produces relief within two hours in 70% to 80% of patients with moderate to severe migraine. Sumatriptan nasal spray has been effective in about 60% of patients after two hours. Oral sumatriptan has been effective in about 50% to 60% of patients with acute migraine after two hours, and in about 70% after four hours (CM Perry and A Markham, Drugs 1998; 55:889).

Four other triptan tablet formulations have been approved by the FDA: **zolmitriptan** *(Zomig)*, **naratriptan** *(Amerge)*, **rizatriptan** *(Maxalt)* and **almotriptan** *(Axert)*. Rizatriptan and zolmitriptan are also available in formulations that dissolve on the tongue *(Maxalt-MLT, Zomig ZMT)*. In one study, almotriptan was as effective as sumatriptan and caused less chest pain (SS Colman et al, Clin Ther 2001; 23:127). Frovatriptan *(Frovelan)* and eletriptan *(Relpax)* may be available soon. Rizatriptan may have a slightly more rapid onset of action than oral sumatriptan (P Tfelt-Hansen, Neurology 2000; 55 suppl 2:S19). Naratriptan, which has a longer half-life, appears to have a slower onset of action and a lower initial response rate. The rate of recurrence of migraine within 24 hours after treatment with a triptan is generally 30% to 40%; it is slightly lower with naratriptan (NT Mathew et al, Neurology 1997; 49:1485).

Adverse Effects – A burning sensation at the injection site is common with subcutaneous sumatriptan. Tingling, flushing, dizziness, drowsiness, fatigue, and a feeling of heaviness, tightness or pressure in the chest may occur with all triptans, but more commonly with injectable sumatriptan. Angina, myocardial infarction, cardiac arrhythmia and death have occurred rarely with these drugs. Both ergots and triptans are contraindicated in patients with coronary or other arterial disease.

Drug Interactions — A triptan or ergotamine-containing drug should not be used within 24 hours after another triptan or ergot because vasoconstriction could be additive. A "serotonin syndrome" of weakness, hyperreflexia and incoordination has occurred rarely in patients taking a selective serotonin reuptake inhibitor (SSRI) with a triptan (RT Jaffe and STH Sokolov, Acta Psychiatr Scand 1997; 95:551). All triptans except naratriptan are contraindicated in patients taking an MAO-A inhibitor or within two weeks of stopping one. Propranolol (*Inderal*, and others) increases serum concentrations of rizatriptan and zolmitriptan (*The Medical Letter Handbook of Adverse Drug Interactions*, 2001, page 437).

PROPHYLAXIS — Patients with frequent or severe disabling migraine headaches, those who cannot take vasoconstrictors and those refractory to acute treatment may benefit from prophylaxis. Menstrual or other predictable migraine attacks may sometimes be prevented by a brief course of an NSAID, ergotamine or a triptan, taken for several days before and during the first few days of menstruation (C Newman et al, Headache 2001; 41:248).

For continuous prophylaxis, **beta-adrenergic blocking agents** are used most commonly. Propranolol and timolol are the only beta-blockers approved by the FDA for this indication. Metoprolol (*Lopressor*, and others), nadolol (*Corgard*, and others) and atenolol (*Tenormin*, and others) have also been effective in preventing migraine, according to Medical Letter consultants. All beta-blockers can cause fatigue, exercise intolerance, depression and orthostatic hypotension, and in the short term may aggravate heart failure. All are contraindicated in patients with asthma.

The antiepileptic drug **valproate** *(Depakote; Depakote ER)* has been effective in decreasing migraine frequency and is approved by the FDA for prevention of migraine. Its effectiveness was equal to that of propranolol in one study (RG Kaniecki, Arch Neurol 1997; 54:1141). *Depakote ER*, a 500-mg tablet for once-daily use only, has caused some confusion because *Depakote* which is taken b.i.d. or t.i.d. is also considered a delayed-release formulation and also is available as a 500-mg tablet. Common adverse effects include nausea, weight gain and fatigue. Valproate can cause polycystic ovary syndrome. Taken during pregnancy, it can cause congenital abnormalities such as neural tube defects. Other antiepileptic drugs such as gabapentin *(Neurontin)* and topiramate *(Topamax)* have also been tried for this indication (NT Mathew et al, Headache 2001; 41:119).

Tricyclic antidepressants can prevent migraine in some patients and may be given concurrently with other prophylactic agents, but often cause weight gain. Amitriptyline (*Elavil*, and others) has probably been used more for this purpose than other antidepressants.

Calcium-channel blockers have also been tried for prevention of migraine. Verapamil (*Calan*, and others) has been moderately effective, but is not FDA-approved for this indication.

Methysergide *(Sansert)*, another ergot alkaloid, is effective for prevention of migraine, but may cause weight gain and peripheral edema. Rare serious complications include retroperitoneal, pleuro-pericardial and subendocardial fibrosis. Major vessel constriction, mesenteric vascular fibrosis and small bowel infarction have been reported. These effects may be idiosyncratic or dose related; continuous use for more than six months without a one-month drug holiday is not recommended. Concurrent use with other ergot alkaloids, a triptan, beta-adrenergic blockers, dopamine or a CYP3A4 inhibitor such as erythromycin may increase the risk of arterial spasm and occlusion (*The Medical Letter Handbook of Adverse Drug Interactions*, 2001, page 270). Methysergide should be reserved for severe refractory migraine.

Nonsteroidal anti-inflammatory drugs (NSAIDs), particularly naproxen sodium (*Anaprox*, and others) and flurbiprofen (*Ansaid*, and others), have been used for short term prevention of migraine as well as for aborting acute attacks.

Botulinum toxin – Pericranial injections of botulinum toxin type A *(Botox)* have been reported to be effective for prophylactic treatment of migraine (S Silberstein et al, Headache 2000; 40:445).

SOME DRUGS FOR PREVENTION OF MIGRAINE

Drug	Usual Dosage	Cost[1]
Beta blockers		
Propranolol – average generic price	80 to 240 mg/day, divided bid, tid or qid	$ 10.80
Inderal (Wyeth-Ayerst)		44.40
Timolol – average generic price	10 to 15 mg bid	19.80
Blocadren (Merck)		38.40
Antiepileptic drugs		
Divalproex sodium – *Depakote* (Abbott)	250 mg bid or tid	67.80
Depakote ER (Abbott)	500-1000 mg once/day	48.90
Tricyclic antidepressants		
Amitriptyline – average generic price	50-150 mg once/day	7.50
Elavil (Zeneca)		25.80
Calcium channel blockers		
Verapamil – average generic price	80 mg tid or qid	18.00
Calan (Searle)		55.80
Serotonin antagonist		
Methysergide – *Sansert* (Novartis)	4 to 8 mg/day, divided bid or tid[2]	133.80

1. Average cost to the patient for 30 days' treatment with lowest daily dosage based on data from retail pharmacies nationwide provided by Scott-Levin's *Source*™ *Prescription Audit (SPA)*, May 2000 to April 2001.
2. Requires 3- to 4-week drug-free period every 6 months.

CONCLUSION — An analgesic may be effective for treatment of mild to moderate migraine. A triptan or dihydroergotamine is the drug of choice for treatment of moderate to severe migraine headache; the injectable and nasal spray forms of sumatriptan have a faster onset of action than the oral form of sumatriptan or any of the other triptans. A beta-blocker is the best established drug for prevention of migraine attacks, but valproate, gabapentin or topiramate may also be worth trying.

DRUGS FOR PAIN

Three types of analgesic drugs are available: first, non-opioids, including aspirin, other nonsteroidal anti-inflammatory drugs (NSAIDs) and acetaminophen; second, opioids; and third, drugs not usually thought of as analgesics, which act as adjuvants when given with NSAIDs or opioids, or have analgesic activity of their own in some types of pain. Non-opioids can be given concurrently with opioids for an additive analgesic effect.

NON-OPIOID ANALGESICS — The maximum analgesic effect of acetaminophen and aspirin usually occurs with single doses between 650 and 1300 mg. With other NSAIDs, the ceiling effect may be higher. Tolerance does not develop to the analgesic effects of these drugs.

Acetaminophen – Acetaminophen is as effective as aspirin, similar in potency and, in single analgesic doses, has the same time-effect curve. Overdosage with acetaminophen can cause serious or fatal hepatic injury, and some patients, such as alcoholics, people who are fasting and those taking isoniazid, zidovudine (AZT; *Retrovir*) or a barbiturate concurrently, may develop hepatic injury after moderate overdosage or even high therapeutic doses (Medical Letter 1996; 38:55). Most patients, however, can take 4 grams a day with no adverse effects.

Aspirin – Aspirin is effective in most types of pain, including cancer pain. Unlike other NSAIDs, a single therapeutic dose irreversibly inhibits platelet function for the 8- to 10-day lifetime of the platelet, interfering with hemostasis and prolonging bleeding time. A single dose of aspirin can precipitate asthma in aspirin-sensitive patients. Multiple doses can cause gastropathy and salicylate intoxication. In children with varicella or influenza, aspirin can cause Reye's syndrome.

Non-Selective NSAIDs — In single full doses, most of the NSAIDs listed on page 145 are more effective analgesics than full doses of aspirin or acetaminophen, and some have shown equal or greater analgesic effect than usual doses of oral opioid combination products, or even injected opioids. Whether this is also true with repeated doses in chronic pain is less well established. Some patients may respond better to one NSAID than another (WT Beaver in GM Aronoff ed, *Evaluation and Treatment of Chronic Pain*, 3rd ed., Baltimore:Williams & Wilkins, 1999, page 455).

Adverse Effects — The adverse effects of non-selective NSAIDs are qualitatively similar to those of aspirin. They can precipitate asthma and anaphylactoid reactions in aspirin-sensitive patients. Unlike aspirin, however, other non-selective NSAIDs cause reversible inhibition of platelet aggregation; platelet function returns when most of the drug has been eliminated. With chronic use, gastrointestinal bleeding, ulceration and perforation can occur, often without warning. Ibuprofen in doses no higher than 1600 mg/day may be less likely to cause serious gastrointestinal toxicity than aspirin or other non-selective NSAIDs (N Moore et al, Clin Drug Invest 1999; 18:89), but fatal hemorrhage and perforation have occurred with all of these drugs. High doses, prolonged use, previous peptic ulcer, excessive alcohol intake and advanced age increase the risk of these complications.

NSAIDs decrease synthesis of renal vasodilator prostaglandins, decrease renal blood flow, cause fluid retention, and may cause renal failure. Risk factors include old age, congestive heart failure, renal insufficiency, ascites, volume depletion and diuretic therapy. Unlike opioids, NSAIDs have no potential for abuse; physical dependence on these drugs has not been reported.

Selective COX-2 Inhibitors — Celecoxib *(Celebrex* — Medical Letter 1999; 41:11 and 28) and rofecoxib (*Vioxx* — Medical Letter 1999; 41:59) appear to cause fewer episodes of serious GI toxicity than non-selective NSAIDs (FE Silverstein et al, JAMA 2000; 284:1247; C Bombardier et al, N Engl J Med 2000; 343:1520). These selective COX-2 inhibitors do not inhibit platelet aggregation or increase bleeding time, and they may have a prothrombotic effect.

Both celecoxib and rofecoxib, if given with warfarin (*Coumadin,* and others), increase INR and prothrombin time values and may increase the risk of bleeding. Other adverse effects are similar to those of non-selective NSAIDs. Single-dose trials have found celecoxib 100 or 200 mg more effective than placebo but less effective than naproxen sodium 550 mg or ibuprofen 400 mg in oral surgery pain, and the FDA has not approved the drug for analgesic use. Single-dose trials have found rofecoxib 50 mg more effective than placebo and as effective as ibuprofen 400 mg or naproxen sodium 550 mg in oral surgery pain.

Ketorolac – Ketorolac is the only injectable NSAID available for analgesic use in the USA. IM or IV ketorolac has analgesic efficacy comparable to moderate doses of morphine or meperidine, with a somewhat slower onset but a longer duration of action (TH Rainer et al, BMJ 2000; 321:1247). Even with parenteral administration, gastrointestinal bleeding can occur.

OPIOIDS — Propoxyphene, pentazocine, and oral codeine and its congeners in usual doses are no more effective when taken alone than aspirin or acetaminophen. They are usually prescribed in combinations with these drugs to treat moderate or moderately severe pain. Morphine, meperidine, hydromorphone, oxymorphone, methadone, levorphanol, fentanyl and large doses of oxycodone are generally used for more severe pain. Opioids are classified as full agonists, partial agonists and mixed agonist-antagonists. Morphine and the other full agonists, unlike NSAIDs, generally have no ceiling for their analgesic effectiveness except that imposed by adverse effects.

Choice of Opioid – The parenteral full agonists listed in the table on page 148 differ in potency, but they are all equally capable of relieving acute pain if the appropriate dose is used. With codeine and meperidine, however, doses that would be equianalgesic with high doses of other agents would cause unacceptable adverse effects.

Morphine – Morphine is the standard of comparison for strong injectable analgesics. Given orally, morphine is well absorbed but extensively metabolized on the first pass through the liver; sustained-release preparations have a longer duration of action. The drug can also be given rectally (N Babul et al, J Clin Pharmacol 1998; 38:74). Morphine has no greater dependence liability than equally effective doses of any other full agonist.

Meperidine – Meperidine has a more rapid onset of action than morphine, but it is irritating to tissues and shorter acting. Repeated doses of the drug lead to accumulation of normeperidine, a toxic metabolite with a 15- to 20-hour half-life that can cause dysphoria, irritability, tremors, myoclonus and, occasionally, seizures, particularly with large repeated doses or decreased renal function. Meperidine should be used only for short-term treatment of acute pain (American Pain Society, *Principles of Analgesic Use in the Treatment of Acute Pain and Cancer Pain*, 4th ed, Glenview, Illinois: American Pain Society, 1999). In patients taking a monoamine oxidase (MAO) inhibitor, meperidine can cause severe encephalopathy and death (*The Medical Letter Handbook of Adverse Drug Interactions*, 2001, page 349).

Methadone and Levorphanol – Methadone and sometimes levorphanol are used orally to relieve pain in patients with chronic pain. Since the plasma half-life of methadone is 24 to 36 hours and that of levorphanol is 12 to 16 hours, repeated doses of either can lead to accumulation and central-nervous-system depression, particularly in elderly or debilitated patients.

Tramadol – An oral opioid agonist that also blocks reuptake of norepinephrine and serotonin, tramadol is marketed for treatment of moderate to moderately severe pain. Its effectiveness is comparable to that of combinations of aspirin or acetaminophen with codeine or propoxyphene. Seizures have been reported with tramadol; patients with a history of seizures and those concomitantly taking an antidepressant, an MAO inhibitor or an antipsychotic drug may be at increased risk. Tramadol is not scheduled as a controlled substance, but opioid-type dependence has occurred.

Fentanyl – Fentanyl is available for parenteral, transdermal and oral transmucosal use. One oral transmucosal formulation *(Actiq)*, a fentanyl lozenge on a handle, is used for treatment of break-through pain in cancer patients already taking strong opioids. It is available in 200- to 1,600-microgram strengths. The appropriate dose is determined by starting with the 200-mcg dose and titrating upward; there is no apparent relationship between the total daily dose of opioids and the dose of transmucosal fentanyl required to manage the breakthrough pain. Adverse effects are typical of strong opioids; patients and caregivers must be cautioned that a single fentanyl lozenge, which resembles a lollipop, can be fatal to a small child.

Partial Agonists and Mixed Agonist/Antagonists – The partial agonist buprenorphine is similar to the mixed agonist/antagonists pentazocine, butorphanol and nalbuphine. All of these drugs have a ceiling on their analgesic effect equivalent to moderate doses of opioids. All can precipitate withdrawal symptoms in patients physically dependent on full agonists. All are less likely than full agonists to cause dependence, but none is free of dependence liability. Only pentazocine is available for oral use and only in combination products. Dependence and abuse have been a problem with use of butorphanol nasal spray for treatment of migraine.

Tolerance to Opioids – Tolerance is common with chronic use of opioids; the patient first notices a shorter duration of analgesia and then a decrease in the effectiveness of each dose. Tolerance can be delayed by using low doses and giving nonopioid analgesics concomitantly. Tolerance to most of the adverse effects of opioids, including respiratory and CNS depression, develops at least as rapidly as tolerance to the analgesic effect. Tolerance, therefore, can usually be surmounted and adequate analgesia restored by increasing the dose. Cross-tolerance exists among all of the full agonists, but it is not complete, and switching to another opioid, starting with half or less of the customary equianalgesic dose, may be helpful.

Dependence – Patients who take strong opioids will develop physical dependence with abstinence symptoms if the drug is discontinued suddenly or an opioid antagonist is given. Clinically significant dependence develops only after several weeks of chronic treatment with relatively large doses of morphine-like opioids. Patients who take opioids for acute pain or cancer pain rarely experience euphoria and even more rarely develop psychological dependence or addiction to the mood-altering effects of opioids.

Adverse Effects – Sedation, dizziness, nausea, vomiting, itching and constipation are the most common adverse effects of opioids; respiratory depression is the most serious. Opioid-induced sedation can be ameliorated by giving small oral doses of dextroamphetamine or methylphenidate in the morning and early afternoon (E Bruera et al, Pain 1992; 50:75). Tolerance usually develops rapidly to the sedative and emetic effect of these drugs, but not to constipation; a stool stimulant or stool softener should be started early in treatment. In one study, transdermal fentanyl caused less sedation and less constipation than sustained-release oral morphine (S Ahmedzhai and D Brooks, J Pain Symptom Manage 1997; 13:254).

In patients with chronic obstructive pulmonary disease, cor pulmonale, decreased respiratory reserve or pre-existing respiratory depression, even usual doses of opioids, including the mixed agonist/antagonists, may decrease respiratory drive and cause apnea. Although patients without pulmonary disease who take opioids chronically are often tolerant to the respiratory depressant effect, opioid-naive acute-pain patients are far more susceptible and therefore must be closely monitored. The addition of general anesthetics, phenothiazines, sedative-hypnotics such as benzodiazepines and barbiturates, tricyclic antidepressants or other CNS depressants increases the risk.

Dosage – Opioid dose requirements vary widely from one patient to another. For most strong opioids, the dose should be increased until adverse effects occur before switching to another opioid. Once the optimal dose that will provide adequate analgesia, hopefully for at least four hours, has been established by titration, it should generally be given for chronic pain on a schedule, with the provision that the patient can refuse a dose if not in pain. "By-the-clock" administration of analgesics is much more effective than waiting for severe pain to return before giving the next dose and may decrease total dosage. An order for a supplementary opioid dose between regular doses should be available as a rescue for breakthrough pain. Patient-controlled analgesia (PCA), given intravenously, subcutaneously or by other routes, is widely used now (Medical Letter 1989; 31:104; NI Cherny, CA Cancer J Clin 2000; 50:70).

ADJUVANT ANALGESICS — Antidepressants and anticonvulsants are the mainstay of therapy for a variety of neuropathic pain syndromes (WS Kingery, Pain 1997; 73:123; SH Sindrup and TS Jensen, Pain 1999; 83:389). Neuropathic pain may be less responsive to opioids than nociceptive pain (P Dellemijn, Pain 1999; 80:453).

Antidepressants – Tricyclic antidepressants such as amitriptyline and imipramine can relieve many types of neuropathic pain, including diabetic neuropathy, postherpetic neuralgia, polyneuropathy, and nerve injury or infiltration with cancer (RL Barkin and J Fawcett, Am J Ther 2000; 7:31). Analgesic efficacy often occurs at lower doses than those used to treat depression. Newer antidepressants have also been effective in some patients with chronic pain (A Ansari, Harvard Rev Psychiatry 2000; 7:257). Venlafaxine *(Effexor)* has been reported to be effective in neuropathic pain (TP Enggaard et al, Clin Pharmacol Ther 2001; 69:245; JE Sumpton and DE Moulin, Ann Pharmacother 2001; 35:557).

Anticonvulsants – Carbamazepine, phenytoin, sodium valproate or clonazepam can also relieve neuropathic pain (IW Tremont-Lukats et al, Drugs 2000; 60:1029). In controlled trials, gabapentin has been effective in diabetic neuropathy and postherpetic neuralgia, and well tolerated (MA Laird and BE Gidal, Ann Pharmacother 2000; 34:802). Lamotrigine and topiramate may also be effective (ZH Bajwa et al, Neurology 1999; 52:1917; PM Simpson et al, Neurology 2000; 54:2115). Lamotrigine has been reported to be moderately effective for central poststroke pain (K Vestergaard et al, Neurology 2001; 56:184).

Caffeine in doses of 65 to 200 mg may enhance the analgesic effect of acetaminophen, aspirin or ibuprofen. **Hydroxyzine** in doses of 25 to 50 mg may add to the analgesic effect of opioids in postoperative and cancer pain while reducing the incidence of nausea and vomiting. **Corticosteroids** can produce analgesia in some patients with inflammatory diseases or tumor infiltration of nerves.

NON-OPIOID ANALGESICS

Drug	Usual analgesic dose	Dose interval	Maximum daily dosage	Comments
Acetamin-ophen (*Tylenol*, others)	PO: 500-1000 mg	q4-6h	4000 mg	As effective as aspirin; 1000 mg more effective than 650 mg in some patients; duration of action usually 4 hours
Salicylates				
Aspirin (many manufacturers)	PO: 500-1000 mg	q4-6h	4000 mg	Duration of action after single doses usually 4 hours
Choline magnesium trisalicylate (*Trilisate*, others)	PO: 1000-1500 mg	q8-12h	3000 mg	Effectiveness compared to aspirin not clear; onset of analgesia probably slower; less gastropathy and impairment of platelet function
Diflunisal (*Dolobid*, others)	PO: 1000 mg initial then 500 mg	q8-12h	1500 mg	500 mg superior to 650 mg of aspirin or acetaminophen, with longer duration
Some Non-Selective NSAIDs				
Diclofenac potassium (*Cataflam*)	PO: 50 mg	q8h	150 mg	Comparable to aspirin with longer duration; available with misoprostol (*Arthrotec*) to decrease GI toxicity
Etodolac (*Lodine*, others)	PO: 200-400 mg	q6-8h	1200 mg	200 mg comparable and 400 mg possibly superior to 650 mg of aspirin

Drug	Usual analgesic dose	Dose interval	Maximum daily dosage	Comments
Fenoprofen (*Nalfon*, others)	PO: 200 mg	q4-6h	1200 mg	Comparable to aspirin; contraindicated in patients with impaired renal function
Ibuprofen (*Motrin*, others)	PO: 400 mg	q4-6h	2400 mg	200 mg equal to 650 mg of aspirin or acetaminophen, 400 mg superior with longer duration; 400 mg comparable to acetaminophen/codeine combination
OTC (*Advil*, *Nuprin*, others)	PO: 200-400 mg	q4-6h	1200 mg	
Ketoprofen (*Orudis*, others)	PO: 25-75 mg	q6-8h	300 mg	12.5 mg comparable to ibuprofen 200 mg; 25 mg comparable to ibuprofen 400 mg and superior to 650 mg of aspirin; 50 mg superior to acetaminophen/ codeine combination
OTC (*Actron*, *Orudis-KT*)	PO: 12.5-25 mg	q4-6h	75 mg	
Ketorolac (*Toradol*, others)	Patients <65 yrs IM or IV: 30 mg Patients ≥65 yrs IM or IV: 15 mg	q6h	120 mg	Comparable to 12 mg IM morphine with longer duration; use should be limited to 5 days; can be given as a single IM dose of 60 mg (<65 yrs) or 30 mg (>65 yrs)
		q6h	60 mg	
	PO: 10 mg	q4-6h	40 mg	10 mg comparable to aspirin or acetaminophen; 20 mg comparable to ibuprofen 400 mg
Meclofenamate	PO: 50-100 mg	q4-6h	400 mg	Comparable to aspirin; approved for dysmenorrhea
Mefenamic acid (*Ponstel*)	PO: 500 mg initial then 250 mg	q6h	1250 mg	Comparable to aspirin but more effective in dysmenorrhea; duration of use not to exceed 1 week

Drug	Usual analgesic dose	Dose interval	Maximum daily dosage	Comments
Naproxen (*Naprosyn*, others)	PO: 500 mg initial then 250 mg OR 500 mg	q6-8h q12h	1250 mg first day then 1000 mg	250 mg probably comparable to 650 mg of aspirin with longer duration; 500 mg superior to 650 mg of aspirin
Naproxen sodium (*Anaprox*, others)	PO: 550 mg initial then 275 mg OR 550 mg	q6-8h q12h	1375 mg first day then 1100 mg	275 mg comparable to 650 mg of aspirin with longer duration; 550 mg superior to 650 mg of aspirin with longer duration
OTC (*Aleve*, others)	PO: 220 or 440 mg initial, then 220 mg	q8-12h	660 mg	440 mg comparable to 400 mg of ibuprofen with longer duration
Selective COX-2 Inhibitors				
Celecoxib (*Celebrex*)	PO: 100-200 mg	q12h	400 mg	Analgesic indication not approved by FDA; more effective than placebo but less effective than full doses of naproxen or ibuprofen
Rofecoxib (*Vioxx*)	PO: 50mg	q24h	50 mg	Efficacy similar to 400 mg ibuprofen or 550 mg naproxen sodium

OPIOID ANALGESICS

Drug	IM dose[1]	IM duration (hours)[2]	Starting oral dose[3]	Comments
Agonists related to morphine				
Morphine	10 mg	3-6	20-60 mg	Available as 8-12h sustained-release tablets (MS-Contin, Oramorph-SR), 12-24h sustained-release capsules (Kadian), and as suppository
Hydromorphone (Dilaudid, others)	1.3 mg	3-5	4-8 mg	Available as high potency injectable (Dilaudid-HP) and as suppository
Oxymorphone (Numorphan)	1.1 mg	3-5	—	Available as suppository
Heroin[4]	4 mg	3-5	—	Adverse effects and dependence liability same as morphine
Agonists related to codeine				
Codeine	130 mg	3-5	30-60 mg	60 mg PO equivalent to 650 mg of aspirin or acetaminophen; usually used orally in combinations with these drugs; some patients resistant to analgesic effect
Dihydrocodeine (Synalgos-DC; DHCplus)	—	—	32 mg	Available only in combination with aspirin or acetaminophen
Hydrocodone (Vicodin, others)	—	—	5-10 mg	10 mg PO equivalent to codeine 60-80 mg PO; available only in combinations with acetaminophen, aspirin, or ibuprofen
Oxycodone (Percocet, others)	—	—	5 mg	10 mg PO equivalent to codeine 90 mg PO; available in combinations, as 5-mg tablets and capsules, as 12-h sustained-release tablets (OxyContin), and oral solution

Drug	IM dose[1]	IM duration (hours)[2]	Starting oral dose[3]	Comments
Synthetic opioid agonists				
Meperidine (*Demerol*, others)	75 mg	2-4	50 mg	More rapid onset of action than morphine, but irritating to tissues IM; toxic metabolite with long half-life causes CNS excitation and convulsions
Fentanyl (*Sublimaze*)	0.1 mg	1-2	—	Transdermal patch (*Duragesic*) for chronic pain releases fentanyl over 72 hours, possibly with less constipation than morphine; oral transmucosal lozenges on a handle are *Actiq* for breakthrough pain and *Oralet* for preanesthetic use
Methadone (*Dolophine*, others)	10 mg	4-6	10-20 mg	Long half-life; risk of CNS depression with repeated use. Dosage reduction often necessary after 24 to 36 hours.
Propoxyphene HCl (*Darvon*, others)	—	—	65 mg	65 mg of HCl or 100 mg of napsylate PO equivalent to codeine 32 mg
Propoxyphene napsylate (*Darvon-N*, others)	—	—	100 mg	PO; available in combinations with acetaminophen or aspirin; convulsions and cardiotoxicity have occurred
Levorphanol (*Levo-Dromoran*, others)	2 mg	4-6	2-4 mg	Long half-life; risk of CNS depression with repeated use

Drug	IM dose[1]	IM duration (hours)[2]	Starting oral dose[3]	Comments
Tramadol (Ultram)	—	—	50-100 mg	50 mg equivalent to codeine 60 mg; 100 mg comparable to aspirin 650 mg plus codeine 60 mg; maximum dose 400 mg/day

Partial agonists and mixed agonist/antagonists

Drug	IM dose[1]	IM duration (hours)[2]	Starting oral dose[3]	Comments
Buprenorphine (Buprenex, others)	0.4 mg	4-6	—	Partial agonist; virtually no psychotomimetic effects; sublingual preparation[4] effective
Pentazocine (Talwin, Talacen)	60 mg	2-4	50 mg	Mixed agonist/antagonist; 50 mg PO equivalent to codeine 60 mg PO; very irritating to tissues; psychotomimetic effects; available in combinations with acetaminophen, aspirin or naloxone (to discourage abuse)
Butorphanol (Stadol)	2 mg	3-6	—	Mixed agonist/antagonist; nasal spray (Stadol NS) comparable to IM injection
Nalbuphine (Nubain, others)	12 mg	3-6	—	Mixed agonist/antagonist; less psychotomimetic effects than pentazocine

1. Equivalent to 10 mg of IM morphine. Much larger doses may be needed after development of tolerance.
2. With an optimal dose established by titration.
3. These drugs are usually given q4-6h, but the duration of action varies with different doses and different patients, and the schedule should be established by titration.
4. Not available for clinical use in USA.

TREATMENT OF PARKINSON'S DISEASE

New drugs for treatment of Parkinson's disease continue to become available to supplement or ameliorate the effects of levodopa. In addition, new neurosurgical approaches are under investigation for treatment of the later stages of the disease (RE Gross and AM Lozano, Neurol Research 2000; 22:247; P Krack et al, J Neurol 2000; 247 suppl 2:122).

LEVODOPA AND CARBIDOPA — Parkinson's disease is caused by progressive degeneration of dopamine-containing neurons in the substantia nigra. Dopamine itself cannot be used to treat Parkinson's disease because it does not cross the blood-brain barrier. Levodopa, the immediate precursor of dopamine, can be used because it is decarboxylated to dopamine in both brain and peripheral tissues. To block this reaction in peripheral tissues, levodopa is combined with carbidopa, a peripheral decarboxylase inhibitor. The combination of these two drugs (*Sinemet*, and others) is the most effective treatment available for symptomatic relief of Parkinson's disease.

Limitations – Levodopa is effective for most patients during the first five years of treatment (W Koller et al, Neurology 1999; 53:1012). Later, as the disease progresses, the duration of benefit from each dose may shorten (the "wearing off" effect), and still later some patients develop sudden, unpredictable fluctuations between mobility and immobility (the "on-off" effect). After about five to eight years of levodopa therapy, patients may have either dose-related clinical fluctuations, dose-related dyskinesias (chorea, dystonia) or inadequate response.

Peripheral adverse effects of levodopa include anorexia, nausea and vomiting, and orthostatic hypotension. Central-nervous-system psychiatric adverse effects include vivid dreams, hallucinations, delusions, confusion and sleep disturbance, especially in older patients. Sudden discontinuation or abrupt reduction of levodopa for several days may cause not only a return of parkinsonian symptoms, but also a neuroleptic malignant syndrome with fever, muscle rigidity and changes in mental status.

Dosage – The daily dose range of levodopa is 300 to 2000 mg usually divided into three or four doses, although some patients may require more frequent dosing. Relatively complete inhibition of peripheral dopa decarboxylase requires 75 to 100 mg/day of carbidopa; some patients require doses of up to 200 mg to completely suppress nausea. Carbidopa *(Lodosyn)* is now available alone and can facilitate dose titration. Dietary amino acids can decrease the effectiveness of levodopa, particularly in patients with advanced disease, by competing with the drug for absorption from the intestine and transport into the brain. Therefore, the drug may be more effective if patients take it at least 30 minutes before eating, and some patients may benefit from restricting daily protein intake until the evening meal.

A controlled-release formulation (*Sinemet CR*, and others) is available in two dosages: 25 mg carbidopa with 100 mg of levodopa and 50 mg carbidopa with 200 mg of levodopa. The higher-dose tablet is scored, but the lower-dose tablet is not, so the smallest individual dose is 25/100 mg of carbidopa/levodopa. Due to its sustained serum levels, the controlled-release formulation can be beneficial for patients who have wearing-off effects. A disadvantage is that it has a slower onset of action, so many patients must take a dose of a standard levodopa-carbidopa combination concomitantly, particularly with the first daily dose, in order to produce a benefit as soon as possible. In addition, levodopa-induced dyskinesias may worsen when treatment is switched from the standard formulation.

Switching to the controlled-release formulation requires titration for some patients. Because only about 70% of levodopa is absorbed from this formulation, the dosage needs to be about 30% higher than the standard combination to achieve a comparable effect. Some clinicians use the controlled-release formulation instead of the standard combination when introducing the drug, starting with 25/100 mg b.i.d. or t.i.d. and increasing gradually to 50/200 mg b.i.d., t.i.d. or q.i.d.

Whether the dosage and duration of levodopa use aggravate Parkinson's disease or simply reflect disease progression is unclear. Levodopa has been implicated as a source of free radicals and potentially could accelerate nigral cell degeneration, but there is no clear evidence that the drug causes neurotoxicity in humans (Y Agid et al, Lancet 1998; 351:851). Nevertheless, because of long-term motor complications, most experts advise beginning levodopa only when symptoms limit function.

SELEGILINE *(Eldepryl,* **and others)** — Another drug widely used to treat Parkinson's disease is selegiline, also known as deprenyl, an irreversible inhibitor of monoamine oxidase type B (MAO-B). Some clinicians begin treatment with selegiline as soon as the diagnosis has been made, reserving levodopa until symptoms become disabling. Treatment with selegiline in early Parkinson's disease before levodopa is introduced can delay the need for levodopa for up to six to nine months. There is no convincing evidence that selegiline slows progression of the disease and it has only a mild effect on symptoms. Since selegiline is metabolized to methamphetamine and amphetamine, it is usually not given late in the day to avoid causing insomnia. The usual dosage is 5 mg twice daily at breakfast and lunch. Many experts believe, however, that 5 mg of selegiline may be as useful as 10 mg in patients with fluctuating Parkinson's disease taking levodopa, and prescribe only one tablet daily (JP Hubble et al, Clin Neuropharmacol 1993; 16:83).

Nausea and orthostatic hypotension may occur with selegiline. At recommended doses, unlike MAO-A inhibitors used for treatment of depression, it generally does not cause hypertension after ingestion of tyramine-rich foods or with concomitant levodopa therapy. The drug may rarely cause toxic interactions with tricyclic antidepressants such as amitryptiline (*Elavil*, and others), selective serotonin reuptake inhibitors (SSRIs) such as fluoxetine *(Prozac)*, and with meperidine (*Demerol*, and others) (*The Medical Letter Handbook of Adverse Drug Interactions*, 2001, page 348). Because selegiline inhibits catabolism and presynaptic reuptake of dopamine in the brain, it can potentiate the effect of levodopa and increase levodopa adverse effects, particularly dyskinesia and psychosis in elderly patients.

DOPAMINE AGONISTS — Dopamine agonists have less antiparkinson effect than levodopa, but are less likely to cause dyskinesias and have a longer duration of action. Used as an adjunct to levodopa in advanced disease, they may contribute to clinical improvement while permitting a reduction in levodopa dosage. Two ergot-derivative dopamine agonists, bromocriptine *(Parlodel)* and pergolide *(Permax)*, are marketed in the USA mainly for adjunctive treatment (with levodopa). Because of its relatively low potency and high cost, bromocriptine is seldom used. A similar drug, lisuride, is available in some other countries. Cabergoline *(Dostinex* – Medical Letter 1997; 39:58), another long-acting ergot dopamine agonist that has been effective in treating advanced Parkinson's disease, has not been marketed in the United States for this indication.

The strategy of using dopamine agonists early as monotherapy or in combination with levodopa to delay long-term levodopa complications is gaining wider acceptance (CW Olanow et al, Neurology 2001; 56 suppl 5:S1). A recent European study demonstrated the efficacy of pergolide in early monotherapy (P Barone et al, Neurology 1999; 53:573). Two non-ergot dopamine agonists, pramipexole *(Mirapex)* and ropinirole *(ReQuip* – Medical Letter 1997; 39:109), are used for treatment of both early (as monotherapy) and advanced disease (with levodopa) (D Lambert and CH Waters, Drugs Aging 2000; 16:55).

Apomorphine, a potent non-ergot dopamine agonist injected subcutaneously or administered intranasally can rapidly reverse the sudden "off" state seen in some patients with advanced Parkinson's disease after long-term levodopa therapy, but is not available in the United States (W Poewe and GK Wenning, Mov Disord 2000; 15:789). Apomorphine causes emesis, but oral domperidone *(Motilium)*, a dopamine antagonist available in Canada but not in the USA, or the antiemetic trimethobenzamide *(Tigan)*, either started two or three days before treatment blocks the emetic effect. A novel sublingual preparation of apomorphine shows promise in treating advanced or fluctuating Parkinson's disease, but requires more clinical trials (W Ondo et al, Clin Neuropharmacol 1999; 22:1).

Dopamine agonists can cause nausea, somnolence and postural hypotension, which may limit their use. The dosage of pergolide is 0.05 mg per day for the first three days, then increasing slowly to 1.5 to 3 mg per day, divided t.i.d. Pramipexole is available in 0.125-, 0.25-, 0.5-, 1-, and 1.5-mg tablets and should be started at 0.125 mg t.i.d. and gradually increased to 0.75 mg t.i.d. over four to six weeks. Further increases should be slower, up to a maximum daily dosage of 4.5 mg. Ropinirole is available in 0.25-, 0.5-, 1-, 2-, 4-, and 5-mg tablets and should be started at 0.25 mg t.i.d. with a slow increase of 0.25- or 0.5 mg per dose each week, up to 3 mg t.i.d. Many patients will need to continue gradually increasing the dose to a maximum of 8 mg t.i.d. The starting dosage of bromocriptine is 1.25 mg daily for the first three days, which then can be increased slowly to 15 to 30 mg per day, divided b.i.d. or t.i.d. with meals.

When used in combination with levodopa, dopamine agonists can potentiate dyskinesias; as the dopamine agonist dosage increases, the levodopa dosage may have to be decreased. Even used alone or in low doses, dopamine agonists can cause confusion and toxic psychosis, particularly in elderly patients. Recently, dopamine agonists taken with levodopa have been reported to cause sudden sleep attacks; patients with Parkinson's disease who drive should be made aware of this uncommon but serious effect (S Frucht et al, Neurology 1999; 52:1908; JJ Ferreira et al, Lancet 2000; 355:1333).

Peripheral dopaminergic effects, such as nausea, can be blocked by domperidone or trimethobenzamide (RB Dewey et al, Mov Disord 1998; 13:782). Some ergot-type effects such as erythromelalgia, edema, pain and digital spasms in the extremities also occur rarely with either ergot or non-ergot dopamine agonists. Pleural effusions causing sudden onset of shortness of breath and/or cough, which have occurred rarely with ergot derivatives, are reversible if the drug is stopped, but permanent fibrotic pulmonary changes and retroperitoneal fibrosis have been reported.

CATECHOL-O-METHYLTRANSFERASE INHIBITORS — Levodopa is metabolized by two enzymes, dopa decarboxylase and catechol-O-methyltransferase (COMT). Used in combination with levodopa-carbidopa, drugs that inhibit peripheral or intestinal activity of COMT prolong the half-life of levodopa and decrease parkinsonian disability and the amount of "off" time, but increase dyskinesias, which may require a reduction in levodopa dosage for control (MC Kurth et al, Neurology 1997; 48:81). Tolcapone *(Tasmar)* is a COMT inhibitor currently marketed in the USA for use as an adjunct to levodopa in patients with severe motor fluctuations (Medical Letter 1998; 40:60). It has caused fatal hepatotoxicity (F Assal et al, Lancet 1998; 352:958) and has been taken off the market in Europe, but is still available in the USA. Monitoring of serum aminotransferase activity is recommended every two weeks; patients who do not respond within three weeks should discontinue the drug.

Another COMT inhibitor, entacapone (*Comtan* – Medical Letter 2000; 42:7) has a much shorter half-life than tolcapone, and must be taken with each dose of levodopa (Parkinson Study Group, Ann Neurol 1997; 42:747). Hepatic toxicity has not been reported with entacapone. Adverse effects that occur with both COMT inhibitors include dyskinesia, nausea, diarrhea (worse with tolcapone) and urine discoloration (worse with entacapone) (S Kaakkola, Drugs 2000; 59:1233). Since these drugs are used in combination with levodopa, the levodopa dose may have to be decreased in patients who develop dyskinesias or hallucinations.

ANTICHOLINERGICS — In Parkinson's disease, the decreased activity of dopamine makes the excitatory effects of acetylcholine more pronounced. Before levodopa, anticholinergic agents were the only drugs available to treat Parkinson's disease, and are still useful in some patients, especially for treatment of tremor and drooling. Although not as effective as levodopa or dopamine agonists, they may have an additive therapeutic effect. Adverse effects of anticholinergic drugs include dry mouth, constipation, urinary retention and aggravation of glaucoma. Central-nervous-system adverse effects including impaired memory, confusion and hallucinations are particularly severe in elderly patients. Anticholinergics available in the USA include trihexyphenidyl (*Artane*, and others), benztropine (*Cogentin*, and others), procyclidine *(Kemadrin)*, and biperiden *(Akineton)*. Ethopropazine *(Parsitan)* is available in Canada. Antihistamines such as diphenhydramine (*Benadryl*, and others) also have anticholinergic effects and may be useful for patients who cannot tolerate the more potent anticholinergics. Abrupt discontinuation of any of these drugs can cause severe exacerbation of symptoms.

AMANTADINE — Amantadine (*Symmetrel*, and others), an antiviral drug, acts as an antagonist at N-methyl-D-aspartate (NMDA) receptors. Its precise mechanism of action in Parkinson's disease is unknown. In a dosage of 100 mg b.i.d., it has been used alone to treat early Parkinson's disease, or as an adjunct in later stages. Amantadine at an average dose of 350 mg/day has been effective in decreasing dyskinesias and motor fluctuations (L Verhagen Metman et al, Neurology 1998; 50:1323). Some patients may not respond, but the drug should be taken for about two weeks before deciding it is ineffective. Nausea, dizziness, insomnia, confusion, hallucinations, ankle edema and livedo reticularis can occur. Amantadine is excreted primarily unchanged in urine; the dosage must be decreased for patients with renal dysfunction. High serum concentrations of amantadine cause severe psychosis. Amantadine and anticholinergics may have additive adverse effects on mental function. Withdrawal of amantadine may cause severe exacerbation of parkinsonian symptoms or neuroleptic malignant syndrome and acute delirium (SA Factor et al, Neurology 1998; 50:1456).

ANTIDEPRESSANTS — Depression commonly accompanies Parkinson's disease and if present, must be treated if the patient is to benefit adequately from antiparkinson drugs. A tricyclic antidepressant or a selective serotonin reuptake inhibitor (SSRI) can be effective. These drugs may also help the sleep abnormalities commonly found in Parkinson's disease. Both worsening of Parkinson's symptoms and reduction in levodopa-induced dyskinesias have been reported with an SSRI. Non-selective MAO inhibitors and irreversible MAO-A inhibitors should not be used because they can cause marked swings in blood pressure in patients taking levodopa. Pramipexole *(Mirapex)* may be helpful for treatment of major depression in patients with Parkinson's disease (MH Corrigan, Depression Anxiety 2000; 11:58). Electroconvulsive therapy (ECT) may alleviate refractory major depression and improve the underlying parkinsonian symptoms (C Moellentine et al, J Neuropsychiatry Clin Neurosci 1998; 10:187).

ATYPICAL ANTIPSYCHOTICS — Clozapine *(Clozaril)* is an antipsychotic drug that does not cause drug-induced parkinsonism and is particularly useful in controlling psychosis associated with levodopa or dopamine agonists in patients with Parkinson's disease (Parkinson Study Group, N Engl J Med 1999; 340:757). Much lower doses of clozapine than those usually needed to treat schizophrenia (6.25 to 50 mg/day versus 300 to 900 mg/day) are effective in levodopa-induced psychosis. Drowsiness is a common adverse effect. The dose is 6.25 or 12.5 mg at bedtime, which can be increased gradually until psychosis is controlled. The drug has also been used to suppress tremor and dyskinesias in patients with Parkinson's disease (U Bonuccelli et al, Neurology 1997; 49:1587; RM Trosch et al, Mov Disord 1998; 13:377). Because clozapine has caused agranulocytosis in 0.6% of patients, weekly blood counts are necessary for the first six months, and biweekly thereafter.

Quetiapine *(Seroquel* – Medical Letter 1997; 39:117), which does not cause agranulocytosis and does not have anticholinergic effects, is now often considered the drug of first choice for treating drug-induced psychosis in Parkinson's disease (JH Friedman and SA Factor, Mov Disord 2000; 15:201). Some Medical Letter consultants, however, believe it is not as effective as clozapine, and there are no published controlled trials comparing the two. Olanzapine *(Zyprexa* – Medical Letter 1997; 39:5), an antipsychotic related to clozapine, does not require blood counts and has been tried for treatment of psychosis in patients with Parkinson's disease; however, many patients treated with olanzapine have had worsening of their parkinsonism (CG Goetz et al, Neurology 2000; 55:789; IH Richard and J Nutt, Neurology 2000; 55:748). Risperidone

(Risperdal), which has potent dopamine D_2 receptor blocking activity, is not usually recommended because it tends to make parkinsonian symptoms worse (MJ Byerly et al, Drugs Aging 2001; 18:45).

SURGICAL TREATMENT — Surgery should generally be reserved for patients with tremor that is refractory to medical treatment or for those with major dyskinesias or clinical fluctuations on levodopa (LI Golbe, Lancet 1998; 351:999). Surgery does not help Parkinson's disease patients who are unresponsive to levodopa.

Several surgical techniques have been tried (P Krack, J Neurol 2000; 247 suppl 2:122). Unilateral ablation of the ventral intermediate nucleus of the thalamus can abolish contralateral tremor in up to 80% of patients, with serious neurological complications occurring in less than 10%. In some patients, improvement has been sustained for more than 10 years. Complications occur more frequently when tremor is severe bilaterally, requiring bilateral ablation. Thalamic procedures are not effective in controlling symptoms of Parkinson's disease other than tremor. Pallidotomy, ablation of the posteroventral portion of the globus pallidus, appears to be effective in controlling dyskinesias, and unilateral pallidotomy, for reasons not yet understood, appears to control some bilateral dyskinesias. Pallidotomy also helps to control bradykinesia, rigidity, tremor and ambulatory difficulties (EC Lai et al, Neurology 2000; 55:1218; J Fine et al, N Engl J Med 2000; 342:1708).

High-frequency electrical stimulation from implanted electrodes in the ventral intermediate nucleus of the thalamus has been reported to control contralateral tremor and possibly levodopa-induced dyskinesias. Deep brain stimulation of the internal globus pallidus has been reported to be effective in improving "on" time, dyskinesias, motor function and activities of daily living. Bilateral deep brain stimulation of the subthalamic nucleus appears to be at least as effective as thalamic stimulation in controlling parkinsonian tremor, although no comparative studies have been published. Bilateral stimulation improves symptoms besides tremor and, compared to pallidal stimulation, has allowed greater post-operative reduction in levodopa dosage. Despite a more complex process for programming the electrical stimulator, subthalamic nucleus stimulation appears to be the most promising surgical technique to date for the treatment of Parkinson's disease (P Pollak, Mov Disord 2000; 15 suppl 3:8).

In both ablative and electrode stimulator operations, adverse effects have included intracranial hemorrhage, hemiparesis, infection, confusion, behavioral changes, attention/cognitive deficits and dysarthria.

In theory, transplantation of dopaminergic cells from human embryonic brain tissue could decrease the severity of disease and permit use of lower doses of levodopa (P Piccini et al, Ann Neurol 2000; 48:689). Follow-up in a large, double-blind US study found that despite improvement at one year in some patients, continuous irreversible dyskinesias developed in 15% of patients during the second year (CR Freed et al, N Engl J Med 2001; 344:710). Newer transplantation techniques under investigation use porcine nigral implants, stem cell implants and genetically engineered cells. Survival and function of dopaminergic neurons may be enhanced by the addition of neurotrophic factors. A new class of oral drugs, nonimmunosuppressive immunophilin ligands, induce dopaminergic nerve terminal branching and sprouting in the denervated striatum in mice, and are being studied in humans (LC Costantini et al, Neurobiol Disease 1998; 5:97).

CONCLUSION — Levodopa combined with carbidopa remains the most effective symptomatic treatment for Parkinson's disease, but many clinicians withhold it early in the disease in an attempt to delay the limitations and complications of long-term use. Dopamine agonists, the next most effective drugs after levodopa in decreasing the symptoms of Parkinson's disease, can be used alone before the introduction of levodopa, or as an adjunct to levodopa. Addition of a peripherally-acting COMT inhibitor to levodopa can reduce motor fluctuations in patients with advanced disease.

DRUGS FOR PARKINSON'S DISEASE

Drug	Usual daily dosage	Cost*
CARBIDOPA/LEVODOPA		
Immediate-release	300 to 2000 mg	
10 mg carbidopa/100 mg levodopa	levodopa, divided	
average generic price		$ 33.30
Sinemet (DuPont)		65.70
25 mg carbidopa/100 mg levodopa		
average generic price		36.00
Sinemet		72.90
25 mg carbidopa/250 mg levodopa		
average generic price		41.40
Sinemet		93.60
Controlled-release	200 to 2200 mg	
25 mg carbidopa/100 mg levodopa	levodopa, divided	
average generic price		73.80
Sinemet CR		86.40
50 mg carbidopa/200 mg levodopa		
average generic price		136.80
Sinemet CR		161.10
DOPAMINE AGONISTS		
Bromocriptine	15 to 30 mg divided	
average generic price	bid or tid	240.30
Parlodel (Novartis)		295.20
Pergolide – *Permax*	1.5 to 3 mg divided	197.70
(Athena Neurosciences)	bid or tid	
Pramipexole – *Mirapex*	0.5 to 1.5 mg tid	175.50
(Pharmacia)		
Ropinirole – *ReQuip*	3 to 5 mg tid	178.20
(GlaxoSmithKline)		
COMT INHIBITORS		
Entacapone – *Comtan* (Novartis)	144.90	
600 to 800 mg divided		
tid or qid		
Tolcapone – *Tasmar* (Roche)	100 mg tid	175.50
OTHER DRUGS		
Selegiline – average generic price (tabs)	5 mg bid at breakfast	78.60
Eldepryl (Somerset)	and lunch	153.00
Amantadine – average generic price	100 mg bid	18.60
Symmetrel (Endo)		64.80
Carbidopa – *Lodosyn* (DuPont)	25 mg tid or qid	51.30

* Average cost to the patient for 30 days' treatment with the lowest recommended dosage, or 3 tablets daily of a levodopa formulation, based on data from retail pharmacies nationwide provided by Scott-Levin's *Source*™ *Prescription Audit* (SPA), May 2000 to April 2001.

DRUGS FOR PREVENTION AND TREATMENT OF POSTMENOPAUSAL OSTEOPOROSIS

Many drugs are now marketed for prevention and treatment of postmenopausal osteoporosis. All regimens should include an adequate intake of calcium and vitamin D.

Drug	FDA-Approved Indication	Dosage	Cost[1]
ESTROGENS[2]	Prevention		
Estradiol, transdermal			
average generic price		15.5 cm^2 patch weekly (0.05 mg/day)	$ 23.44
Climara (Berlex)		6.5 cm^2 patch weekly (0.025 mg/day)	26.96
Estraderm (Novartis)		10 cm^2 patch 2/week (0.05 mg/day)	26.16
Vivelle (Novartis)		11 cm^2 patch 2/week (0.0375 mg/day)	26.24
Estradiol, micronized – average generic price		0.5 mg PO daily	7.84
Estrace (Apothecon)			12.60
Gynodiol (Fielding)			8.40
Esterified estrogens		0.3 mg PO daily	
Estratab (Solvay)			14.28
Menest (Monarch)			8.12
Estropipate – generic		0.75 mg PO daily	10.08
Ogen (Pharmacia & Upjohn)			21.56
Conjugated equine estrogens			
Premarin (Wyeth-Ayerst)		0.625 mg PO daily	17.92
ESTROGEN COMBINATIONS[2]			
Estradiol/norgestimate			
Ortho-Prefest (Ortho-McNeil)		1 mg daily x 3 days, followed by 1 mg/ 0.09 mg daily x 3 days, repeated	24.92

1. Average cost to the patient for 28 days' treatment, based on data from retail pharmacies nationwide provided by Scott-Levin's *Source*™ *Prescription Audit (SPA)*, May 2000 to April 2001.
2. For a woman with an intact uterus, a progestin must be added to estrogen therapy. Oral estrogens are usually given continuously or in a cyclic regimen.

Drug	FDA-Approved Indication	Dosage	Cost[1]
Estradiol/norethindrone acetate			
Activella (Pharmacia & Upjohn)		1 mg/0.5 mg daily	$ 27.44
femhrt (Parke-Davis)		5 µg/1 mg daily	23.80
Conjugated equine estrogens/ medroxyprogesterone			
Premphase (Wyeth-Ayerst)		0.625 mg PO daily days 1-14, then 0.625 mg/5 mg PO daily days 15-28	26.32
Prempro (Wyeth-Ayerst)		0.625 mg/2.5 mg PO daily	28.28
BISPHOSPHONATES			
Alendronate – *Fosamax*	Prevention	5 mg PO daily	57.40
(Merck)		or 35 mg PO weekly	60.00
	Treatment	10 mg PO daily	57.12
		or 70 mg PO weekly	59.60
Risedronate – *Actonel*	Prevention,	5 mg PO daily	51.24
(Procter & Gamble)	Treatment		
SELECTIVE ESTROGEN RECEPTOR MODULATOR			
Raloxifene – *Evista* (Lilly)	Prevention, Treatment	60 mg daily	58.24
CALCITONIN	Treatment		
Calcitonin-salmon – average generic price		100 IU SC or IM every other day	238.14
Miacalcin Injection (Novartis)		100 IU SC or IM every other day	259.84
Miacalcin Nasal Spray (Novartis)		200 IU intranasal daily	63.74[3]

3. Cost of two 2-ml bottles with at least 14 doses each based on AWP listings in *Drug Topics Red Book Update*, June 2001.

BONE DENSITOMETRY — Typically, the need for drug therapy is established by bone densitometry (Medical Letter 1996; 38:103), which is generally reported in terms of standard deviations (SD) from mean values in young adults (T score) and age-matched controls (Z score). The World Health Organization has defined normal bone mineral density (BMD) for women as a value within one SD of the young adult mean. Values 1 to 2.5 SD below the mean are defined as osteopenia, and those more than 2.5 SD below the mean are defined as osteoporosis. The risk of fracture increases with age and with each SD below the young adult mean.

CALCIUM AND VITAMIN D — In adults more than 65 years old, a high calcium intake combined with vitamin D can increase BMD and reduce the incidence of fractures. The Institute of Medicine of the National Academy of Sciences recommends a daily intake of 800 mg of calcium for children 4 to 8 years old, 1300 mg for children 9 to 18, 1000 mg for adults 19 to 50, including pregnant and lactating women, and 1200 mg for those over the age of 50, including those taking estrogen (Medical Letter 2000; 42:29). Vitamin D is necessary for optimal calcium absorption. The recommended minimum daily requirement of vitamin D is 200 IU for adults younger than 50 years old, 400 IU for adults 51 to 70 years old and 600 IU for those over 70. Some experts recommend a vitamin D intake of 800 IU/day for all adults (RD Utiger, N Engl J Med 1998; 338:828).

ESTROGEN — Lack of estrogen after menopause is associated with rapid bone loss due to increased osteoclast activity and bone resorption. A three-year, prospective double-blind trial in 875 postmenopausal women (mean age 56) found that hormone replacement therapy increased spine BMD by 3.5% to 5.0% and hip BMD by 1.7%, compared to an average loss of 1.8% and 1.7% of spine and hip BMD with placebo (The Writing Group for the PEPI Trial, JAMA 1996; 276:1389). When estrogen is discontinued, rapid bone loss resumes.

Retrospective studies of estrogen in women with established osteoporosis have reported a decrease in the incidence of spine and hip fractures (NIH Consensus Development Panel, JAMA 2001; 285:785). No large prospective studies have shown that estrogen prevents fractures. In one 12-month double-blind trial in 75 women with established osteoporosis, women using transdermal estrogen had 8 vertebral fractures, compared to 20 in women on placebo (EG Lufkin et al, Ann Intern Med 1992; 117:1). One cohort study also found a reduced risk of fracture in women taking estrogen, including those who were more than 75 years old (JA Cauley et al, Ann Intern Med 1995; 122:9).

Adverse Effects – Adverse effects of estrogen therapy include bloating, breast tenderness and uterine bleeding. Women who have an intact uterus must also take a progestin to avoid an increased risk of endometrial cancer. Long-term estrogen use increases the risk of thromboembolism and might increase the risk of breast cancer (WC Willett et al, JAMA 2000; 283:534).

BISPHOSPHONATES — These nonhormonal agents with a high affinity for bone inhibit osteoclast function, decreasing bone resorption.

Alendronate (Medical Letter 1996; 38:1), an oral bisphosphonate, is approved by the FDA for prevention (5 mg daily) and treatment (10 mg daily) of osteoporosis. Once-weekly use of 35 mg for prevention and 70 mg for treatment has also been approved; it appears to be equally effective and may be better tolerated (Medical Letter 2001; 43:26).

A prospective study of alendronate 5 mg/day given for two years to 1174 postmenopausal women without osteoporosis who were less than 60 years old found 3.5% and 1.9% increases in BMD at the lumbar spine and hip with the drug, and decreases in BMD with placebo (D Hosking et al, N Engl J Med 1998; 338:485). In more than 4000 postmenopausal women aged 54 to 81 years with low bone mass but no history of vertebral fracture, alendronate 5 mg daily for two years followed by 10 mg daily for two more years increased BMD at all sites and decreased the number of symptomatic fractures from 312 with placebo to 272 with the drug; this decrease was not statistically significant (SR Cummings et al, JAMA 1998; 280:2077). A third prospective trial in more than 2000 postmenopausal women with low bone mass and at least one vertebral fracture at baseline found that over 36 months new symptomatic fractures at any site occurred in 183 women taking placebo and in 139 taking alendronate. Hip fractures occurred in 22 women on placebo and 11 taking alendronate (DM Black et al, Lancet 1996; 348:1535). In men with osteoporosis alendronate has also increased BMD and prevented vertebral fractures and decreases in height (E Orwoll et al, N Engl J Med 2000; 343:604).

Risedronate – Risedronate, another oral bisphosphonate, is approved by the FDA for prevention and treatment of osteoporosis in postmenopausal women, and may also become available in a once-weekly formulation. In a two-year study in 111 postmenopausal women (mean age 51) with normal lumbar spine BMD, patients taking 5 mg per day showed a 1.4% gain in spine BMD and a 2.6% increase at the femoral trochanter, compared to decreases at both sites with placebo. One year after stopping treatment, lumbar spine BMD was 2.3% lower than baseline in the patients who had taken daily risedronate and 5.6% lower in those who had taken placebo (L Mortensen et al, J Clin Endocrinol Metab 1998; 83:396).

A three-year trial in about 1000 postmenopausal women (average age 69) with low bone mass and at least one vertebral fracture found that the incidence of new vertebral fractures was 11% with 5 mg of risedronate daily and 16% with placebo (ST Harris et al, JAMA 1999; 282:1344). A three-year controlled trial in more than 5000 high-risk elderly women with osteoporosis found that risedronate 2.5 or 5 mg daily decreased the incidence of hip fracture compared to placebo (MR McClung et al, N Engl J Med 2001; 344:333).

Adverse Effects — Alendronate and risedronate can cause heartburn, esophageal irritation, esophagitis, abdominal pain, diarrhea and other adverse gastrointestinal effects. Alendronate taken once weekly may be less irritating. Calcium supplements taken at the same time may interfere with absorption of bisphosphonates. To ensure adequate absorption and avoid esophageal injury, either alendronate or risedronate must be taken after an overnight fast, while in an upright position, along with 8 oz of plain water. After taking the drug, the patient must consume nothing else for at least 30 minutes and avoid lying down. The long-term effects of these drugs are unknown.

Etidronate — Although not approved by the FDA for use in postmenopausal osteoporosis, etidronate *(Didronel)*, another oral bisphosphonate, has been used by some clinicians for two weeks every three months in a cyclic regimen (PD Miller et al, Am J Med 1997; 103:468).

RALOXIFENE — Raloxifene (Medical Letter 1998; 40:29) is a selective estrogen receptor modulator (SERM) with estrogen-like effects on bone and cardiovascular tissue and antiestrogen effects on the uterus and breast. One clinical trial showed a marked reduction in the risk of breast cancer in postmenopausal women with osteoporosis taking raloxifene (SR Cummings et al, JAMA 1999; 281:2189). In another trial, 601 postmenopausal women (average age 55) without osteoporosis took raloxifene or placebo daily for two years. The women receiving active treatment had statistically significant increases in lumbar spine and hip BMD, while bone mass decreased in those taking placebo (PD Delmas, N Engl J Med 1997; 337:1641).

In 7705 postmenopausal women with established osteoporosis, lumbar spine and femoral neck BMD after three years were 2.1% to 2.7% higher with raloxifene than with placebo. Among women taking 60 mg and 120 mg of raloxifene, 6.6% and 5.4% had new vertebral fractures, compared to 10.1% in the placebo group. The risk of nonvertebral fractures, however, was about the same with raloxifene as with placebo (B Ettinger et al, JAMA 1999; 282:637).

Adverse Effects – Hot flashes and leg cramps can occur in patients taking raloxifene. Like estrogens, raloxifene increases the risk of thromboembolic events. Whether raloxifene could, like tamoxifen (*Nolvadex*, and others), increase the risk of uterine cancer remains to be established.

CALCITONIN — This peptide hormone decreases bone resorption by inhibiting osteoclast function, and may also have an analgesic effect. A controlled five-year trial in 1200 women with osteoporosis found new vertebral fractures in 51 of 287 (18%) receiving a 200 IU dose of salmon calcitonin nasal spray once daily and in 70 of 270 (26%) receiving a placebo. Fracture reductions with a higher dose of 400 IU were not statistically significant (CH Chestnut III et al, Am J Med 2000; 109:267). This study has been criticized because the investigators were aware of bone density results during the study and 59% of the women not only did not complete the study, but also were lost to follow-up (SR Cummings and RD Chapurlat, Am J Med 2000; 109:330). The effect of calcitonin on sites other than the spine has been equivocal.

Adverse Effects – Subcutaneous calcitonin injection has been used for nearly 30 years without serious adverse effects. Nausea and flushing occur commonly. Rhinitis and occasional epistaxis have occurred with the intranasal preparation.

PARATHYROID HORMONE — Parathyroid hormone (PTH) increases bone density by stimulating bone formation. A prospective placebo-controlled trial in 1637 women (average age 70) with postmenopausal osteoporosis and at least one vertebral fracture found about one third the incidence of vertebral fractures (4% to 5% vs 14%) and about half the incidence of non-vertebral fractures (3% vs 6%) in women who gave themselves subcutaneous injections of recombinant human PTH 20 or 40 µg once daily for 21 months (RM Neer et al, N Engl J Med 2001; 344:1434). Adverse effects included nausea, headache, dizziness and leg cramps. In rats, high doses of recombinant parathyroid hormone have induced osteosclerosis and osteogenic sarcoma. Parathyroid hormone is not yet commercially available; it is under development as teriparatide (*Forteo* – Lilly).

COMBINATION THERAPY — In one double-blind trial, 425 postmenopausal women with low BMD were treated with placebo, alendronate 10 mg, estrogen replacement or combined estrogen-alendronate therapy for two years. The mean increase in spine BMD was greatest with combination therapy (8.3% compared to a 6% gain in both monotherapy groups, and an 0.6% loss with placebo). The increases in proximal femoral bone density with alendronate, estrogen, alendronate-estrogen and placebo were 4.0%, 3.4%, 4.7% and 0.3%, respectively (HG Bone et al, J Clin Endocrinol Metab 2000; 85:720). Combinations of estrogen and calcitonin have also had beneficial additive effects on BMD. Whether combination therapy leads to a greater reduction in the risk of fractures remains to be established.

STATINS — Some **HMG-CoA reductase inhibitors (statins)** have marked osteogenic effects in rodents (G Mundy et al, Science 1999; 286:1946). Observational studies have suggested that statin treatment reduces fracture risk in elderly patients (KA Chan et al, Lancet 2000; 355:2185; CR Meier et al, JAMA 2000; 283:3205; PS Wang et al, JAMA 2000; 283:3211), but other have offered no support for this hypothesis (IC Reid et al, Lancet 2001; 357:507; T-P van Staa et al, JAMA 2001; 285:1850).

CONCLUSION — Alendronate, risedronate and raloxifene are effective in preventing vertebral fractures in postmenopausal women with osteoporosis. Estrogen may also be effective in preventing vertebral fractures, but large prospective controlled trials are lacking. Only alendronate and risedronate have been shown to prevent hip fractures. The benefits of calcitonin in preventing fractures are less well established. Once-daily injections of recombinant human parathyroid hormone decrease the incidence of fractures in women with established osteoporosis.